A Caregiver's Guide to Communication Problems from Brain Injury or Disease

A Johns Hopkins Press Health Book

A CAREGIVER'S GUIDE TO

Communication Problems *from* Brain Injury or Disease

EDITED BY

Barbara O'Connor Wells, PhD, CCC–SLP
AND Connie K. Porcaro, PhD, CCC–SLP

 Johns Hopkins University Press
Baltimore

Note to the reader: This book is not meant to substitute for medical care, and treatment should not be based solely on its contents. Instead, treatment must be developed in a dialogue between the individual and his or her physician. The book has been written to help with that dialogue.

Johns Hopkins University Press
2715 North Charles Street
Baltimore, Maryland 21218-4363
www.press.jhu.edu

Library of Congress Cataloging-in-Publication Data

Names: O'Connor Wells, Barbara, 1972– editor. | Porcaro, Connie K.,
    1964– editor.
Title: A caregiver's guide to communication problems from brain injury or dis-
    ease / edited by Barbara O'Connor Wells, PhD, CCC-SLP, Connie K. Porcaro,
    PhD, CCC-SLP.
Description: Baltimore : Johns Hopkins University Press, 2022. | Series: A Johns
    Hopkins press health book | Includes bibliographical references and index.
Identifiers: LCCN 2021006368 | ISBN 9781421442549 (hardcover) |
    ISBN 9781421442556 (paperback) | ISBN 9781421442563 (ebook)
Subjects: LCSH: Brain—Diseases—Handbooks, manuals, etc. | Brain—Diseases—
    Patients—Care—Handbooks, manuals, etc. | People with mental disabilities—
    Care—Handbooks, manuals, etc.
Classification: LCC RC386 .C37 2022 | DDC 616.8—dc23
LC record available at https://lccn.loc.gov/2021006368

A catalog record for this book is available from the British Library.

Chapter illustrations are from Adobe Stock inspired by drawings by Alexa Keintz. Illustrations in the appendixes are from iStock.com.

Special discounts are available for bulk purchases of this book. For more information, please contact Special Sales at specialsales@jh.edu.

To all patients and families we have had the blessing of working with throughout our careers. Your journey was the inspiration. We hope this book will help, inspire, and encourage those who follow.

Contents

Contributors

Marissa A. Barrera, PhD, MSCS, CCC-SLP

Program Director and Associate Professor, Yeshiva University

Frederick DiCarlo, EdD, CCC-SLP

Associate Professor, Nova Southeastern University

Lea Kaploun, PhD, CCC-SLP

Associate Professor, Nova Southeastern University

Elizabeth Roberts, PhD, CCC-SLP

Associate Professor, Nova Southeastern University

Teresa Signorelli Pisano, PhD, CCC-SLP

Visiting Scholar (Retired), The Graduate Center of the
City University of New York

Acknowledgments

We could not have taken the journey of editing and writing this book without the help and support of so many people. Words cannot express our gratitude for the role you played in helping us put our vision into print. Our thanks:

To the editorial team at Johns Hopkins University Press, for working so hard to put our manuscript into print. Special thanks to Joe Rusko, whose Christmas Eve 2019 email started this whole process, and to Adelene Jane Medrano, for supporting us through all the editorial steps.

To Dr. Michelle McRoy-Higgins, for graciously sharing her ideas on book proposals and how to navigate the publishing world. Her book *Time to Talk: What You Need to Know About Your Child's Speech and Language Development* inspired us to create a book for caregivers of persons with adult communication, memory, and swallowing disorders.

To Dr. Jackie Hinckley for advising and supporting us in the development of this book, providing her expertise as a chapter reviewer, and connecting us with caregivers and professional contacts at various stages in this process.

To Dr. Audrey Holland, a guru in adult language disorders and our professional idol, who read an earlier version of the book in its entirety and gave us her honest and helpful feedback.

To our contributors, who put their heart and soul into their respective chapters and met deadlines with patience and professionalism. We truly enjoyed taking this journey with you:

Dr. Elizabeth Roberts, who took inspiration from her grandparents and great-grandmother, as well as the many patients with dementia she has worked with over her professional career, to form a chapter filled with helpful ideas to meet the challenges of dementia.

Dr. Frederick DiCarlo, who shared his extensive theater background and passion for the arts, as well as his own clinical infusion of the arts in his professional practice, to give caregivers practical ways to help their loved ones continue to explore and enjoy the world, even with the challenges of communication impairment.

Dr. Lea Kaploun, who brought her substantial teaching experience in counseling and her clinical background in leading caregiver support groups and working with individuals who have communication impairment due to acquired brain injury and degenerative disease, to create her heartfelt and memorable chapter.

Dr. Marissa A. Barrera, who generously shared her extensive and globally renowned knowledge of swallowing disorders in her chapter to assist patients and caregivers in taking a more active role in their health care decisions related to nutrition.

Dr. Teresa Signorelli Pisano, who used her research and clinical background on healthy aging to create our first chapter, allowing readers to identify the normal aging process compared to the impacts of acquired brain injury and degenerative disease.

To Alexa Keintz, who meshed her knowledge of the field of speech-language pathology with her artistic talent to create the simple and informative illustrations that begin each chapter.

To the professionals who were carefully chosen, based on their expertise, to review individual chapters. Thank you for providing useful content and editing suggestions to ensure the reader would be armed with the most meaningful and up-to-date information. These reviewers included Dr. Michelle Bourgeois, Dr. Mario Landera, Dr. John McCarthy, Dr. Luis Riquelme, Dr. Kristy Weissling, and Dr. Christine Williams.

To the caregivers who reviewed individual chapters. We were so honored that you gave of your valuable time and shared your feedback on how the chapter you reviewed was meaningful to you and spoke to your own personal experience and struggles in caring for a loved one with a communication disorder.

And finally, to our beloved families, for your unconditional love, patience, and encouragement on the journey to creating this book. We are blessed beyond measure to have supportive spouses, children, and extended families. We are forever thankful for the greatest cheerleaders of all, our parents, June and Joe O'Connor and Fran and Edward Himrich. We couldn't have done this without you all!

A Caregiver's Guide to Communication Problems from Brain Injury or Disease

Introduction

Barbara O'Connor Wells, PhD, CCC-SLP,
and Connie K. Porcaro, PhD, CCC-SLP

Given advances in modern science and medicine, people are more likely to survive a stroke or live with a degenerative disease, like Parkinson's, for longer than was possible in the past. When a person has an acquired brain injury or degenerative disease, they will probably have deficits that affect multiple areas of communication. For a person who has experienced a stroke, it is common to have speech, language, voice, and swallowing deficits. A person diagnosed with Parkinson's disease, as another example, will often have speech, voice, memory, and swallowing problems. It is crucial for that person and their caregivers to have a comprehensive understanding of what to expect and how to best facilitate communication in all areas affected by their medical diagnosis. We created this book to help educate caregivers about these critical issues. If the examples above resonate with you, and you have struggled to communicate with your loved one, this book will change your life.

In our society, the caregiver's role may be complex and dynamic over time. Depending on the type of acquired brain injury or degenerative disease a person experiences, caregivers can be thrust into a heavy role of dealing with all day-to-day tasks, including communicating for their loved one. In other cases, when a disease progresses

1

more slowly, the caregiver's role may expand over time. A caregiver can wear many hats, including cheerleader, advocate, support system, information gatherer, glue that holds the family together, medication controller, reminder of appointments, errand runner, and grocery shopper. Caregivers may include spouses, adult children, siblings, or health care aides. These individuals work with health care specialists, such as speech-language pathologists, occupational therapists, and physical therapists to reinforce rehabilitation strategies in the home environment. A common goal among all is to assist the person with communication challenges in making compensations and using strategies to help them continue to live a happy, healthy, and fulfilled life.

The goal of this book is to provide you, the caregiver, with useful information and strategies to address the communication, memory, and swallowing challenges your loved one may be experiencing. It begins with an overview of the healthy aging process, including expected age-related changes in speech, memory, and hearing abilities, to name a few. We present this chapter first, to help readers identify differences between normal healthy aging and the effects of acquired brain injury or degenerative disease. This chapter can also guide the caregiver in navigating their own aging process and how that can affect their caregiver role. Following that, the next several chapters provide user-friendly information on anticipated changes in speech, voice, swallowing, language, and memory from an acquired brain injury or a degenerative disease. While these chapter topics are distinct, a common thread of helpful communication strategies and tips is reinforced in each chapter. We also include a counseling chapter that covers grief, coping, and caring for the patient and you, the caregiver. This chapter acknowledges your struggles in managing the day-to-day challenges related to your loved one's communication, memory, or swallowing issues. The last chapter of this book describes how to incorporate the arts, including your loved one's previous hobbies, interests, and talents, into the rehabilitation or home program.

Each chapter begins with case studies, and we use common questions on the topic of the chapter as subheadings that are easy for readers to follow. In addition, we provide definitions of common medical terms and helpful resources. We believe this organization will allow you to take a more informed and active role in your loved one's care. We are confident this is the all-in-one resource on communication, memory, and swallowing you have been searching for.

We carefully chose the chapter authors, based on their extensive personal and professional experiences in working with many individuals who have communication, memory, and swallowing disorders. As doctoral-level faculty from universities around the United States, the contributors have the skills to teach you, the caregiver, what you need to know about your loved one's communication challenges. In this book, the authors share their personal and clinical experiences in working closely with caregivers and patients. After reading our book, you will have strategies and helpful resources to apply to your own situation of caring for a loved one with a communication disorder. The chapter authors skillfully present real-life case scenarios for each topic area to help you relate to the communication, memory, or swallowing problems your loved one may be experiencing.

A caregiver's need for specific information may change as their loved one improves or declines because of the degenerative disease process or recovery that occurs in the brain. This book allows a reader to spend 10 minutes learning about effective memory strategies for dementia or to take time for a more thorough reading of the entire book to learn about multiple topics. Our book takes caregivers step by step through the rehabilitation process for all deficits related to communication, memory, and swallowing. As a caregiver, you will need to be well informed about the potential changes that may occur in communication, memory, or swallowing. We recommend that you learn as much as you can about your loved one's diagnosis. Begin by finding as many resources as possible, such as books, websites, and medical professionals. Learn the basics about your loved one's acquired brain injury or degenerative disease. You will need to make decisions, and you will have an easier time if you are well educated. Families feel more in control when they have a greater understanding of their loved one's acquired brain injury or degenerative disease. It is also important to realize that you are not alone in your challenges. You will find answers, strength, and comfort in talking to other people who have been in your shoes. Joining a support group will allow you to make connections with those people. This will help you create realistic expectations for the rehabilitative process and the compensations needed for residual deficits. Caregivers will naturally have questions about how they can best facilitate success in communication (speech, language, voice), memory, nutrition, or swallowing for their loved one. You may want to know how to help if your partner's speech is not clear enough to be understood by your grandchildren. You may be looking for ways to help when your mother can't remember how to get home from the mall, or how to change the diet of your uncle to prevent choking. This book provides answers to assist caregivers in dealing with these situations and many more.

To help you learn more about your loved one's challenges, in this next section, we review six causes of acquired brain injury or degenerative disease that can lead to impaired communication, memory, and swallowing. We provide this information so you can better understand what is happening to the brain and nervous system of your loved one. This is not a complete list by any means, so you may need to find additional information elsewhere for diagnoses not covered here. This is an overview to help you get started. It is important to seek more in-depth information, as needed, and under the guidance of your loved one's medical team. Stroke and traumatic brain injury are used here as examples of acquired brain injury. For degenerative diseases, we present examples of dementia, Parkinson's disease, multiple sclerosis, and amyotrophic lateral sclerosis.

What Are Some Important Things to Know about Stroke?

A stroke, also called a cerebrovascular accident (CVA) or "brain attack," is a neurological impairment that affects the arteries leading to and within the brain. According to the American Stroke Association (www.stroke.org), stroke is a leading cause of death and disability in the United States every year. It is also the most common cause of language problems in adults (see chapter 5 for a discussion of aphasia).

What Happens to the Brain When a Person Has a Stroke?

There are two major types of strokes: ischemic and hemorrhagic. Ischemic strokes are more common. This type of stroke involves a blockage of blood flow and oxygen to the brain because of plaque buildup inside the artery in the brain (called *thrombosis*) or a traveling blood clot from somewhere else in the body, such as the heart or lungs (called *embolus*). In ischemic strokes, the areas of the brain that don't get blood flow and oxygen become impaired and no longer function. In hemorrhagic strokes, too much blood accumulates in or surrounds the brain because of a rupture of a blood vessel. As a result of the bleed, necessary oxygen does not reach brain tissue. Also, because of extra blood in or outside the brain, there is added pressure, which further deprives the brain of needed oxygen. According to Cleveland Clinic (2020), brain tissue deprived of blood for even a few minutes can lead to brain cell death. Brain hemorrhage can be caused by a traumatic injury to the brain or conditions like a brain aneurysm. A transient ischemic attack, also called a TIA or "ministroke," is a temporary clot that disrupts the blood flow to the brain.

In a stroke, if an area of the brain doesn't get the necessary blood flow and oxygen, or if there is too much blood to that area, the functions it serves will not work. This can lead to motor and sensory problems, such as paralysis or paresis (weakness) to one side of the body, increased tension (spasticity) of the muscles, fine motor problems (for example, problems with buttoning a shirt, picking up utensils), problems with vision, or difficulties with other sensations, such as touch.

How Does a Stroke Affect Communication, Memory, and Swallowing?

Depending on the area of the brain affected by the stroke, the person may have difficulty with communication that affects how they express themselves or understand language, which is called *aphasia* (see chapter 5). These language problems will probably occur if the stroke involved the middle cerebral artery on the left side of the brain. Some cognitive skills, like attention, memory, and problem solving, may also be affected but are usually seen in strokes that involve the right side of the brain. Speech may be labored, slurred, or difficult to understand, known as either *apraxia of speech* or *dysarthria* (see chapter 2). These speech problems will probably occur if the frontal lobe of the left side of the brain is damaged. A stroke can also cause swallowing problems, known as *dysphagia* (see chapter 4). If the medulla or other brainstem (lower brain) structures are damaged, the swallowing problems may be severe.

What Are Important Things to Know about Traumatic Brain Injury?

Traumatic brain injury, also referred to as TBI, brain injury, or head injury, is damage to the brain that occurs when an outside force acts on the head and brain. According to the Centers for Disease Control and Prevention (CDC, 2020), a TBI can be caused by a bump, blow, or jolt to the head that interrupts how the brain normally works. TBIs can be caused by either a moving object that strikes the head or the head striking a stationary, or nonmoving, object. An example of a moving object striking the head is a gunshot wound or a baseball bat to the head, while the head striking a stationary object is what happens, for example, in a car accident when a person's head hits the steering wheel. A TBI can have devastating consequences to both the person who has the TBI and their family (Family Caregiver Alliance, 2020).

There are two main types of TBI: penetrating, or open, head injury and nonpenetrating, or closed, head injury. In an open head injury, an object tears open the protective layers of the brain (called the *meninges*) and fractures the skull, as happens with a gunshot wound. This type of head injury is less common than a closed head injury and is mostly associated with wartime or military injuries. Nonpenetrating, or closed, head injury occurs when the person's skull and meninges remain intact. There is no opening into the head. The most common causes of all head injuries are falls and motor vehicle crashes.

TBIs can vary in severity, from mild to severe. In mild cases, the person may have only a minor concussion, which we have seen on the rise in sports-related injuries. A mild brain injury will lead to only a brief change in mental status or loss of consciousness and may go undiagnosed and untreated (Family Caregiver Alliance, 2020). According to the CDC (2020), most people with a TBI recover well from symptoms, and most TBIs are mild concussions. Frequent mild TBIs, however, can leave a person susceptible to a more severe TBI at a later time. In severe cases, the person may lose consciousness and be in a coma for an extended period.

There are several risk factors for brain injury (Family Caregiver Alliance, 2020). These include (1) age: TBI is most common among adolescents (ages 15–24) and older adults (75 and older); (2) gender: more common in males than females; (3) substance abuse: history of substance abuse (drugs, alcohol) can leave a person prone to brain injury; (4) personality: persons who are daring risk takers (for example, high-risk sports, competitive sports, motorcycle riders) are more likely to suffer a brain injury than someone who is more cautious and guarded; or (5) prior history of neurological impairment, such as TBI: if a person has a previous history of a neurological impairment, like stroke or previous TBI, it makes their brain vulnerable to another brain injury.

What Happens to the Brain When a Person Has a TBI?

Various primary and secondary injuries can happen as a result of a TBI. Primary injuries are those that happen at the time of the injury. These include things such as abrasions (scratches), lacerations (cuts), or contusions (bruises) to the brain; hemorrhages (bleeding in the brain); diffuse axonal injury (a tearing of brain tissue seen in severe injuries); or skull fractures. Secondary factors, which occur over time, include cerebral edema, or brain swelling. This is caused by excess fluid in or outside the brain that causes brain tissue to swell, either at the main site of the brain injury or at a more distant site in the brain. This swelling puts extra pressure on the brain. The medical team may place a shunt in the brain to drain the excess blood or fluid.

How Does a TBI Affect Communication, Memory, and Swallowing?

Any TBI, whether mild or severe, can lead to problems in speech, language, voice, swallowing, or memory. In addition, it can cause impairments in movement (for example, weakness and impaired balance), sensation (for example, vision, hearing, sensation of touch), or emotional functioning (for example, personality changes or depression). These issues can have lasting effects on the person with the brain injury and their relationships with families and friends (CDC, 2020).

Depending on the area of the brain affected by the TBI, the person may experience voice changes. For example, the person's voice may sound strained and strangled, harsh, or breathy (see chapter 3 for a discussion of voice problems). They may have speech problems, where, because of muscle weakness or spasticity, the speech muscles don't move correctly, and the result is slurred or difficult-to-understand speech (see chapter 2 for a discussion of speech problems). A TBI can also cause cognitive problems, such as shortened attention span, memory difficulties, concentration problems, trouble learning new things, and poor judgment. It can also cause changes in personality, such as difficulty with social skills, inappropriate behavior, trouble controlling one's emotions, increased mood swings, and even depression (CDC, 2020).

Individuals with TBI often have trouble with communication, such as word-finding problems, difficulty participating in conversation, and impaired understanding of abstract concepts, like what the phrase "don't cry over spilled milk" means. They may interrupt the conversational partner and have difficulty with pragmatic functions, like eye contact in conversation (see chapters 5 and 6 for a discussion of communication and cognitive problems). An acquired brain injury can also cause swallowing issues, such as pocketing food in the mouth or choking when eating or drinking (see chapter 4 for a discussion of swallowing problems). After a severe acquired brain injury, a person may have residual complications that cannot be improved with treatment and will require the family and caregivers of the person to make accommodations to the home environment.

What Are Some Important Things to Know about Dementia?

According to the Alzheimer's Association (2021), dementia is a general term for various diseases and conditions characterized by a decline in memory, language, problem-solving, and other thinking skills that affect a person's ability to perform everyday activities. There are several types of dementia and a variety of causes. Alzheimer's disease is the most common cause, accounting for about 60%–80% of all dementia cases (Alzheimer's Association, 2021). Vascular dementia, caused by a history of brain bleeding and blockage (such as multiple strokes), is the second most common type of dementia.

Some risk factors for dementia, include (1) age (more common in older adults, with the risk increasing after age 65); (2) gender (more common among women than men, at a worldwide ratio of 2:1; see Alzheimer's Society, 2021); and (3) family history or genetic predisposition to dementia. No one can change these risk factors. Other risk factors are under a person's control: living a healthy lifestyle, eating a balanced diet, exercising regularly, and keeping our brains active and stimulated can help ward off or reduce the risk of dementia.

Some possible early signs or symptoms of dementia include problems with short-term memory, forgetfulness (such as losing one's belongings or forgetting familiar persons' names), difficulty with common daily tasks, such as preparing meals and paying household bills. Unlike a stroke or TBI, dementia is a progressive degenerative disorder, meaning that the person's symptoms will get worse over time (Alzheimer's Association, 2021).

What Happens to the Brain When a Person Has Dementia?

Dementia is caused by damage to brain cells, which interferes with the ability of these brain cells to communicate with one another. Damage to cells in a specific area of the brain will cause that area to not function properly. A person's thinking, behavior, or movement will be affected, depending on which areas of the brain are impaired.

The brain has many distinct regions responsible for different functions (for example, memory, judgment, and movement). When the brain cells in a specific area of the brain are damaged, that area cannot carry out its functions normally. Each type of dementia is associated with brain cell damage in particular areas of the brain

(Alzheimer's Association, 2021). For example, one of the key deficits in Alzheimer's dementia is problems with memory, which is due to damage to brain cells in an area of the brain called the *hippocampus*, which is an important area in the brain for learning and memory. Persons with Alzheimer's disease also show amyloid plaques (clumps of protein that form in the spaces between nerve cells) and neurofibrillary tangles (knots of brain cells made up of tau protein) on brain imaging. These plaques and tangles damage healthy neurons in the brain and the fibers that connect them. In vascular dementia, there is damage to the blood vessels and white matter areas of the brain (Mayo Clinic, 2019a).

Treatment for dementia depends on the type and cause. For the types that are progressive, such as Alzheimer's dementia, no cure or specific treatment will help prevent the decline or slow the disease progression. Nonetheless, medical professionals caring for a person with dementia will use drug treatments to help improve symptoms (Alzheimer's Association, 2021).

How Does Dementia Affect Communication, Memory, and Swallowing?

Dementia symptoms vary depending on the cause. For some persons, the key deficits will be in the areas of cognition, communication, and personality. These can include (1) memory loss, confusion, and disorientation; (2) difficulty with problem solving and organizing one's thoughts; (3) visual-spatial orientation problems, such as getting lost in a familiar setting; (4) trouble finding words; (5) personality changes; (6) hallucinations; and (7) emotional changes, like anxiety and depression (Mayo Clinic, 2019a). In addition, the person with advancing dementia may develop problems with nutrition and swallowing. Because of the cognitive decline, the person with dementia may lose their appetite, refuse meals, lose weight, "forget" how to swallow (for example, holding food and liquid in their mouth), and develop a condition called *failure to thrive*. This topic of dementia is the focus of chapter 6 of this book.

What Are Important Things to Know about Parkinson's Disease?

Parkinson's disease (PD) is a disorder of specific areas of that brain that slowly gets worse over time. Some key characteristics of PD are tremors in muscles when they are at rest (resting tremor), increased muscle tone that makes the body rigid and stiff, slowness of movement (called *bradykinesia*), and difficulty with balance. All people with PD will experience movement difficulties, and some will also have impaired thinking (dementia). Some individuals are diagnosed with PD before the age of 50, which we call *early onset PD*. The strongest risk factor associated with PD, however, is age, meaning it is more common in older individuals.

What Happens to the Brain When a Person Has Parkinson's Disease?

We have structures that are located deep inside our brain called the *basal ganglia*. These structures help us start our movements and make them smooth. When we reach for a pen on the table, these structures communicate with the muscles that will move our arm to reach out and our fingers to grasp the pen. The basal ganglia also help coordinate changes in our posture. So if the pen was across the table and we had to lean over to reach for it, that coordination takes place between the basal ganglia and other structures and muscle. The basal ganglia also keep us from making involuntary movements. This helps us keep our foot from moving, which might throw off our balance when we are reaching to pick up the pen. The basal ganglia produce a neurotransmitter called dopamine, which sends messages through nerves to muscles. In PD, the basal ganglia do not produce enough dopamine, which decreases the connections between the nerves and muscles. This results in the symptoms discussed earlier, including tremor; slow, small movements; difficulties with posture and walking; and stiffness (American Parkinson Disease Association, 2021).

How Does Parkinson's Disease Affect Communication, Memory, and Swallowing?

The small, slow movements of people with PD can cause speech that may not be easily understood. Many people with PD have very soft voices that are monotone, and they convey little emotion with their words or facial movements. Their voice may sound hoarse or breathy, and they may trail off near the end of a sentence (see chapter 3 for further information on voice issues). Words may sound slurred, and some people with PD will speak slowly, while others speak rapidly and almost sound like they are stuttering (see chapter 2 information on dysarthria). Memory issues do not occur in everyone with PD, but some people experience slow thinking and processing, as well as difficulty with memory. About 40% of those with PD develop dementia (American Parkinson Disease Association, 2021), which is further discussed in chapter 6. The movement issues associated with PD commonly impact a person's ability to swallow safely and may range from mild to severe as the disease progresses. Difficulties might include swallowing certain foods or drinks, coughing or clearing the throat while eating or drinking, and having the sensation that food is getting stuck. See chapter 4 if you want to read more about swallowing difficulties that might relate to PD.

What Are Important Things to Know about Multiple Sclerosis?

Diagnosis of multiple sclerosis (MS) can take place at any age, but the typical age range is between 20 and 50 years. Symptoms of MS commonly include difficulties with balance, walking, vision, and movements (Multiple Sclerosis Association of America, 2017). A relapse may occur where symptoms get worse, followed by a period of remission, when the symptoms lessen. Some individuals have a gradual progression of symptoms with little or no remission.

What Happens to the Brain When a Person Has MS?

The nerves in our body help to move messages to and from our brain. Our nerves have a coating on them that is like the plastic coating on electrical cords that protects the wires inside. We call this coating *myelin*, and it covers most of the nerves in our body. In MS, the myelin is damaged or destroyed. We do not know why this occurs, but we suspect the body's immune system is attacking the person's own tissues (Mayo Clinic, 2020). MS mainly affects nerves in the brain related to vision and those in the spinal cord that help us move our bodies and limbs. Damaged myelin will not allow messages from the brain to get all the way through to muscles, and this can affect movements.

How Does MS Affect Communication, Memory, and Swallowing?

MS can cause communication issues such as slurred speech (called dysarthria, see chapter 2), nasal voice, and low volume (see chapter 3). Weakness in the respiratory system and in the head can cause these issues. MS can result in memory impairment when communication between nerves in the brain breaks down (MS LifeLines, 2019). This will cause difficulty remembering information that was recently heard or learned, as well as losing items (see chapter 6 for more information on memory). Coughing, choking, and difficulty chewing and swallowing can lead to a lack of safe, effective swallowing in individuals with MS. There can also be some loss of sensation in the throat and chest area, which can affect safe swallowing (see chapter 4 for information on swallowing).

What Are Important Things to
Know about Amyotrophic Lateral Sclerosis?

Amyotrophic lateral sclerosis (ALS) is a disease affecting the nerves in the brain and spinal cord, where movement is progressively impaired over time. We commonly call this Lou Gehrig's disease, after the famous New York Yankees baseball player who had ALS and put a face to the disease. Over the course of ALS, there will be serious impairment in the ability to walk, talk, swallow, and breathe. In 2014, fund-raising efforts for ALS resulted in the Ice Bucket Challenge, which greatly increased awareness of and research for this disease.

What Happens to the Brain When a Person Has ALS?

For normal movements to happen, nerves carry messages from the brain to muscles. The nerve cells that move our limbs and body move through the spinal cord in our back to send messages out to the body. The nerve cells that communicate with our head and neck move through the brainstem, which forms the connection between the brain and the spinal cord. When we wave to our friend across the street, the message starts in the brain, and nerves carry the message to the muscles in our arm and hand to wave a friendly "hello." In ALS, the nerve cells deteriorate over time. This causes the muscles in the body to become slowly weaker and waste away (atrophy). At some point, there may be complete paralysis—no movement of muscles at all. This can happen in the muscles that move our arms and legs, but also in those that help us breathe, speak, or swallow.

ALS is not the same in every single person, and there are two different ways this disease can begin. Some people have difficulty initially with movements of their hands, arms, and legs. Remember these muscles receive information from the brain through nerves that travel through the spinal cord. Later, these same individuals will have difficulty with the nerves that communicate with the face and neck, which will cause speech and swallowing difficulties. In some people, ALS affects the face and neck muscles first, followed by the limbs and body. Everyone who has a diagnosis of ALS will have these muscles affected significantly during the disease process, resulting in weakness, muscle atrophy, cramps, and fatigue (Mayo Clinic, 2019b). The person's movements may be stiff and clumsy, and sometimes the muscles twitch. There is a tremendous impact on swallowing and speech. A person may not be able to speak or swallow near the end of the disease process.

How Does ALS Affect Communication, Memory, and Swallowing?

People with ALS have a great deal of difficulty breathing, and this can affect their ability to communicate in normal ways. Their voice can become quiet and nasal (see chapter 3), and their speech is often very slurred (see chapter 2). Eventually, most people with ALS end up using a device to communicate, known as augmentative/alternative communication. Memory issues, even frontotemporal dementia, can occur in some people with ALS (see chapter 6). Chewing and swallowing safely are also impaired over time, and a feeding tube may be needed in some cases to ensure safe intake of food and liquid in individuals with ALS (see chapter 4).

Concluding Thoughts

In this introduction to our book, we present you, the caregiver, with an overview of symptoms that might be noted in acquired brain injury or degenerative disease. It is important to remember that the symptoms described may overlap with the aging process in an older individual. A loved one with a TBI, for example, may also have some normal age-related changes in communication that can easily be confused with disordered symptoms because of brain injury. For this reason, our book begins with the aging process in normal healthy adults. In chapter 1, you will read information that applies to both you and your loved one. From there, you can read the chapters that relate to the communication, memory, or swallowing problems you are dealing with. You may need some chapters now, and some later, as symptoms improve or worsen. There is an old saying that "knowledge is power." Our goal is to arm you, the caregiver, with the knowledge of how to help your loved one with communication, memory, and swallowing challenges. We hope you will feel inspired by this book and will recommend it to others who could benefit from this resource.

REFERENCES

Alzheimer's Association. (2021). *What is dementia?* Retrieved February 2, 2021. https://www.alz.org/alzheimers-dementia/what-is-dementia.

Alzheimer's Society. (2021). *We're here, so how can we help?* Retrieved February 2, 2021. https://www.alzheimers.org.uk/.

American Parkinson Disease Association. (2021). *What is Parkinson's disease?* https://www.apdaparkinson.org/what-is-parkinsons/.

Centers for Disease Control and Prevention (CDC). (2020, August 28). *Traumatic brain injury and concussion.* https://www.cdc.gov/traumatic braininjury/.

Cleveland Clinic. (2020, May 4). *Brain bleed, hemorrhage (intracranial hemorrhage).* https://my.clevelandclinic.org/health/diseases/14480-brain-bleed -hemorrhage-intracranial-hemorrhage.

Family Caregiver Alliance. (2020). *Traumatic brain injury.* https://www .caregiver.org/traumatic-brain-injury.

Mayo Clinic. (2019a, April 19). *Dementia: Symptoms and causes.* https:// www.mayoclinic.org/diseases-conditions/dementia/symptoms-causes /syc-20352013.

Mayo Clinic. (2019b, August 6). *Amyotrophic lateral sclerosis (ALS).* https:// www.mayoclinic.org/diseases-conditions/amyotrophic-lateral-sclerosis /symptoms-causes/syc-20354022.

Mayo Clinic. (2020, June 12). *Multiple sclerosis: Symptoms and causes.* https://www.mayoclinic.org/diseases-conditions/multiple-sclerosis /symptoms-causes/syc-20350269.

MS LifeLines. (2019). *Cognitive issues.* https://www.mslifelines.com/under standing-ms/signs-and-symptoms-of-ms/ms-cognitive-impairment.

Multiple Sclerosis Association of America. (2017, October 31). *MS symptom listing.* https://mymsaa.org/ms-information/symptoms/ms-symptoms/.

RESOURCES

Alzheimer's Association: https://www.alz.org
  What Is Dementia?: https://www.alz.org/alzheimers-dementia/what-is -dementia
Alzheimer's Society: https://www.alzheimers.org.uk
American Parkinson Disease Association: https://www.apdaparkinson.org/
American Stroke Association: https://www.stroke.org
American Stroke Foundation: https://americanstroke.org
Amyotrophic Lateral Sclerosis (ALS) Association: http://www.alsa.org/
Centers for Disease Control and Prevention (CDC): https://www.cdc.gov
  Traumatic Brain Injury and Concussion: https://www.cdc.gov/traumatic braininjury/
Cleveland Clinic: https://my.clevelandclinic.org/
  Brain Bleed, Hemorrhage (Intracranial Hemorrhage): https://my.cleveland clinic.org/health/diseases/14480-brain-bleed-hemorrhage-intracranial-hemorrhage
Family Caregiver Alliance (FCA): https://www.caregiver.org
  Traumatic Brain Injury: https://www.caregiver.org/traumatic-brain-injury
Mayo Clinic: https://www.mayoclinic.org
  Amyotrophic Lateral Sclerosis (ALS): https://www.mayoclinic.org/diseases -conditions/amyotrophic-lateral-sclerosis/symptoms-causes/syc-20354022
  Dementia: https://www.mayoclinic.org/diseases-conditions/dementia /symptoms-causes/syc-20352013
  Multiple Sclerosis: https://www.mayoclinic.org/diseases-conditions /multiple-sclerosis/symptoms-causes/syc-20350269

Vascular Dementia: https://www.mayoclinic.org/diseases-conditions
/vascular-dementia/symptoms-causes/syc-20378793

The Michael J. Fox Foundation for Parkinson's Disease Research: https://
www.michaeljfox.org

MS LifeLines: https://www.mslifelines.com

Multiple Sclerosis Association of America: https://mymsaa.org/

MS Symptom Listing: https://mymsaa.org/ms-information/symptoms
/ms-symptoms/

Multiple Sclerosis Foundation: https://msfocus.org/

National Alliance for Caregiving: https://www.caregiving.org

National Aphasia Association: https://www.aphasia.org/

National Multiple Sclerosis Society: https://www.nationalmssociety.org/

Parkinson's Foundation: https://www.parkinson.org/

Voices of Hope for Aphasia: http://www.vohaphasia.org/

Well Spouse Association: https://www.wellspouse.org

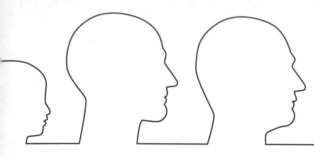

What's Her Name and Where Are My Glasses?

The Ironies of Healthy Aging

Teresa Signorelli Pisano, PhD, CCC-SLP

The art of life lies in a constant readjustment to our surroundings.
Kakuzo Okakura, Japanese scholar

John and Abigail got dressed for dinner. It was their fifty-fifth wedding anniversary. John fastened Abby's brooch to her blouse. Her hands were too stiff to do it. He stopped halfway through to put on reading glasses to see the clasp better.

"John, please don't remove your dentures at the restaurant. I know you think it's funny, but it's not a good example for the kids."

"Yes, Abby. But if Tom tells us one more time what we should do now that we're retired, I may give him a piece of my mind."

"How about you thank him for his concern and suggest our celebration dinner is not the time to talk about it?"

John agreed. He finished dressing and went to the living room to wait with their daughter and her husband, who were driving them to the restaurant. A good 20 minutes passed before Abby joined them.

"Ma, I told you we'd be here at a quarter of 7:00. It's 7:15. How could you not be ready?" their daughter snapped.

"Don't be fresh with your mother, young lady," her father corrected.

"I'm sorry, I just don't want to miss the sunset for pictures."

The daughter was smart enough not to say it was because she didn't want to get home late. It took her parents longer to eat than it used to.

"Dad, you realize you have Mom's pink rhinestone reading glasses on," said the son-in-law.

"Yes, I can't find mine, and we have similar prescriptions. Besides, I think they work well with my suit."

"You're bold, man."

"I'm an old man?!"

"No, BOLD, fearless!"

"Ah, yes, thanks. I'll adjust my hearing aids."

The four arrived at the restaurant 15 minutes later. Abby caught her foot on the stoop leading into the restaurant, and John clasped her elbow to steady her. The hostess brought them to the table on the deck where the rest of the family was waiting. She took a picture of the three generations smiling together. No one would know until later that the youngest grand-daughter had smacked her brother's face as he pulled her hair.

The art of life may lie in how well we adjust to our surroundings, as Okakura suggests above. I would add that it also lies in how well we adjust to aging. Many challenges can develop as we age. This chapter provides an overview of the healthy aging process, mostly related to communication from *physical*, *intellectual*, and *social-emotional* angles. You saw aspects of this in the story above about *John* and *Abby*. Some characteristics of healthy aging, like memory loss, ease of learning, and some communication challenges, overlap with symptoms of genuine disorders and diseases.

It seems strange, but there is a normal decline in skills that comes with age. We optimistically call it healthy aging. There is also decline that comes from degenerative diseases, like Parkinson's disease or

Alzheimer's disease, or from acquired brain injuries, like stroke and head injury from a fall. Several of these are described in the introduction. This can sometimes blur the differences between normal aging and changes that result from a degenerative disease or an acquired brain injury. Understanding these differences is especially important to help ensure that loved ones receive appropriate health care in either case and to assist with early diagnosis and intervention with a degenerative disease or an acquired brain injury.

Areas of human development, like physical, intellectual, and social-emotional development, influence one another. So decline in one area could cause problems in another. An older person who is not as intellectually quick or as physically strong as they used to be, for example, may become depressed over their skill loss. Knowing how these areas change and potentially interact can also help health care professionals make an accurate diagnosis and identify the best treatment options. This can help promote the best quality of life as we age. When one considers the US Census Bureau's (2017) estimate that nearly 48 million older adults make up our population, understanding aging and its impact on communication is important.

Communication is a physical and intellectual (or mental) activity that occurs through expressive and receptive language. Language expression happens when we use words and sentences to organize ideas and then express them physically through speech and writing. We also express our ideas with facial and body gestures. Alternatively, we use language receptively to understand what someone else says, writes, or gestures. To comprehend someone's message, we physically need to hear what they say, read what they print, or see what they gesture. This exchange takes place in a social context with other people. Finally, the communication mechanism, which includes body parts like the mouth and throat, is also used for eating and drinking. Consequently, we have included a chapter on swallowing disorders in this book. This is an area that speech-language pathologists address given our knowledge and training on the parts of the body involved in swallowing, communication, and their related disorders.

Please realize that aging changes are not disorders and are not the same for everyone. We all age in different ways and to different extents. Having good genes is helpful, as is leading a healthy lifestyle. A happy, optimistic outlook can also work wonders in maintaining a healthy body, mind, and disposition through our senior years. Aside from age-related changes, older adults are at increased risk for several degenerative diseases and acquired brain injuries. Although this book is not exhaustive, my knowledgeable colleagues and I have insightful and useful information to help you with your loved one facing communication, cognition, speech, or swallowing challenges. We hope this book can help you foster a better quality of life for you and those you love.

What Are Some Physical Changes That Occur with Healthy Aging?

Let's begin with physical changes, as these are more obvious than others. At least they feel that way to me. First, I address vision and hearing related to language, as well as speech, voice, and swallowing.

Vision

Whatever you may look like, marry a man your own age.
As your beauty fades, so will his eyesight.
Phyllis Diller, comedian

You are reading right now, so why not address vision first? Reading is a visual and an intellectual task. Letters, words, and punctuation marks make up the print we see. When we read, we connect the letter symbols to the sounds related to them. We string these together to make words that have meaning. Punctuation marks also have meaning. Thus, there is a connection with our long-term memory, or knowledge.

We sequence words to form sentences. We hold on to information in the beginning of the sentence while we read the later parts to make sense of it. As a result, our working memory is also important. Working memory is the set of mental activities we use to process and store information over a brief period. Vision is also important to spoken communication, as it helps us understand what we hear. We might, for example, notice facial and body gestures that influence the meaning of spoken speech. If your friend says he is happy to see you and smiles, that tells you one thing. If he says he is happy to see you and rolls his eyes, that tells you something else. Let's hope he smiles.

So what happens as we age? Vision changes throughout adulthood, which can affect how we perform activities in our day-to-day life. You might have noticed a change in your eyesight, for example, when you started holding dinner menus farther and farther away to read. Many of us in middle age and older are familiar with a condition called *presbyopia,* in which it is difficult to see things up close. It's the reason why *John* put on *Abby's* readers. This is a part of normal aging that typically begins in adults around age 40 (Mukamal, 2015). While there is no way to stop or reverse this gradual vision decline, the American Academy of Ophthalmology (AAO, 2015) reports we can correct the condition with glasses, contact lenses, and even surgery.

Owsley's (2016) review of aging vision highlights several age-related deficits that can affect quality of life. She reports, for example, that older adults may have difficulty detecting object borders or patterns. In this case, it might become difficult to see the edges of an unfamiliar set of stairs. Recall that *Abby* caught her foot on the restaurant stoop. Seeing in low light might also become difficult, making it a challenge to drive at night or read a menu in a restaurant with dim lighting. Aging could also affect the time needed to recognize an object or to discriminate objects. Older adults are also at higher risk for certain eye diseases and conditions. The National Eye Institute (2019) reports that the most common age-related eye diseases and conditions include age-related macular degeneration, cataracts, diabetic retinopathy, dry eye, glaucoma, and low vision. Mukamal (2015) also reports that floaters, where you might see small dots or lines, and flashes, where you might see streaks of light, can occur in our visual field as we get older and, sometimes, can lead to blindness.

Phyllis Diller's quotation above tries to turn fading eyesight into a blessing in the face of fading beauty, but it really is not. An early referral to specialists, like ophthalmologists, who are medical doctors, or optometrists, who are eye care professionals, is important when one considers how important vision is to quality of life. Vision problems can also indicate genuine diseases or disorders. Furthermore, having vision corrected can help protect against cognitive decline. Research from Rodgers and Langa (2010), for example, shows that cognitive skill decline is potentially higher in older adults with uncorrected vision. Dentone and Afshari (2019) also note that without vision correction, we could experience eyestrain and headaches. So what can we do? The AAO (2015) suggests that individuals have eye exams every two to four years between the ages of 40 and 54; every one to three years ages 55 to 64; and every one to two years ages 65 and up or as physician recommended. The AAO also proposes good eye hygiene practices, like wearing sunglasses to protect eyes from UV radiation damage, keeping your doctor informed about any family history of eye disease, eating right, avoiding smoking, and controlling blood pressure, cholesterol, and blood sugar.

Hearing

I am at an age where I have to find my
hearing aid to ask where my glasses are.
Robert Orben, comedian

Robert Orben's comment above is another amusing example of the connection between hearing and vision. Oral communication, or speaking, may be what many people think of most when they think of communication. This makes hearing well critical to satisfying wants and needs and connecting with friends and loved ones. Let's also stress that good communication is a safety issue. If you hear "take fifty pills over the week" when the doctor said "fifteen pills," there could be terrible consequences.

Let's review how hearing works. The outer ear funnels sound to the middle ear, where the eardrum vibrates and moves a tiny chain of bones that connect to the inner ear. The inner ear is full of tiny hair cells that respond to different aspects of sound. These cells then send the sound information up to the brain for processing—that is, for making sense of the information so that an individual can hear, or better yet, understand whether it is speech or environmental sounds like a car horn.

The National Institute on Deafness and Other Communication Disorders (NIDCD, 2018) reports that the gradual loss of hearing that occurs with age is one of the most common conditions older adults face. I hope you find comfort being in good company if you or your loved one is hard of hearing. The NIDCD (2018) estimates that 33% of individuals ages 65 to 74 and almost 50% of individuals over age 75 experience hearing loss. With its slow onset, people rarely notice their hearing decline. Friends and loved ones, on the other hand, sometimes painfully do.

One can experience hearing challenges at any of these points in the system. Hearing loss due to aging, called *presbycusis*, is primarily a result of inner ear changes. When the ear's hair cells are not functioning well, the brain receives incomplete information, and this causes comprehension to be poor. While the condition cannot be reversed, it can improve with hearing aids and strategies to improve communication. Not all hearing challenges in older adults occur because of how the ear captures and sends sounds to the brain. Sometimes, the ear is working just fine. Instead, the source of the trouble may be the brain processing information less efficiently as we age. So, unfortunately, listening comprehension can decline because of age-related changes in the ear and in the brain.

Brain-based hearing challenges can begin in our forties. As Koehnke, Lister, and Wambacq (2015) note, processing speed can decline. Problems can also be an issue of how well the brain combines information coming from your right and left ears. These brain-based processing challenges might cause difficulty understanding conversation, especially when there is some background noise, as in a crowded room. This might cause problems identifying the location a sound comes from. Attention and memory changes in aging can also play a role in these problems. It might become difficult to focus on what a speaker says or hold information in memory sufficiently to understand it well.

There's a joke I once heard about three senior citizens chatting outside. The first says something like, "Windy, isn't it?" The second replies, "No, it's Thursday," and the third responds, "So am I. Let's get a drink." This misunderstanding among friends because of poor hearing in a casual interaction is humorous. When miscommunication takes place regularly, however, among family, friends, or coworkers, it can be a source of frustration, anxiety, and maybe even danger. Communication partners may repeat what they say and speak louder. Individuals with hearing loss may have trouble understanding short phrases and following conversation. This can be an irritation that limits social participation and affects quality of life. We did not notice frustration when *John* misheard his son-in-law, but it can happen.

These social and emotional factors are likely why Helen Keller profoundly said, "Blindness cuts us off from things, but deafness cuts us off from people." In a survey of the literature on hearing loss, the elderly, and quality of life, Ciorba and colleagues (2012) found there is real impact. They reported that older adults with hearing loss can have emotional reactions such as loneliness, depression, and anger.

They can also show changes in behavior, such as bluffing, blaming, or withdrawing.

Hearing loss due to normal aging can be difficult to estimate, because conditions like diabetes and high blood pressure, and even certain medications, can cause hearing loss. Following a stroke or other brain diseases, individuals may develop a language disorder called *aphasia*. They may have trouble understanding speech, which can look similar to hearing loss. (See chapter 5 for more information on aphasia.) Hearing loss can also occur because of overexposure to noise. This is a concern, as noise pollution—noise at irritating and even damaging levels—is more prevalent in our culture than many people realize. If you must raise your voice for someone to hear you over sounds like street traffic, music, and beeps and buzzes in the workplace, you are in noise pollution.

Since hearing trouble can also indicate more than normal age-related decline, we should have regular hearing screenings as we age. Protecting your hearing from excessive noise and getting helpful devices like hearing aids, if needed, are also wise. As with vision, there is a relationship between hearing and cognition. Research, such as that of Lin and colleagues (2013), suggests that cognitive skills can decline faster in individuals with hearing loss compared to those without. They also found an increased risk of dementia with hearing loss (see chapter 6).

For more information on hearing, I encourage you to visit the American Speech-Language and Hearing Association (ASHA) website (www.asha.org). Members of this association include speech-language pathologists, audiologists, and scientists and students in these related disciplines in the United States. An audiologist is the health care professional to go to for preventing and assessing disorders related to hearing and balance. Your inner ear is involved in your sense of balance. Audiologists also provide treatment, such as hearing aid fitting and use. Speech-language pathologists assess, diagnose, and treat speech, language, and swallowing challenges. This includes working with individuals with hearing loss, to help them use strategies to improve communication.

Speech Mechanism, Part I: Articulation, Voice, and Fluency

Speech has power. Words do not fade.
What starts out as a sound, ends in a deed.
Abraham Joshua Herschel, theologian and philosopher

Speech has power. Speaking is a critical way we meet our wants and needs. You are actually speaking silently in your head while you are reading here, so why not review speech production? To speak, we exhale air from our lungs, which makes our vocal cords (folds) vibrate, creating our voice. The vibrating air gets filtered by our lips, teeth, tongue, jaw, soft palate, throat, and nose to create the sounds that then form words. Some air vibrates in our nasal cavities, contributing to the sound quality of our voice. You can see these structures in appendix A. The last aspect of speech production is fluency, which means the ease and flow with which we produce sounds and words.

Hooper and Cralidis (2009), in their review of the research on normal speech changes in older adults, report potential changes across the different speech-production mechanisms. In terms of lung function, for example, older adults may produce fewer words per breath and speak with decreased loudness. Vocal fold changes may occur with aging that result in declining voice loudness and quality. Common changes in voice quality may include hoarseness, scratchiness, or breathiness when too much air escapes; voice breaks; or the sound of the voice suddenly becoming too high.

While there may be some aging challenges, other aspects of speech production seem to be relatively more resistant to aging. The resonance quality of the voice, involving vibration in the nasal areas, for example, remains fairly intact. The clarity and precision of speech in older adults typically remains good, even with some challenges from dentures. *John* seemed to have no problem with his. The same is true for speech fluency, or smoothness. For more information on speech disorders and what you can do for them, see chapter 2, which addresses the muscular disorder dysarthria and the motor-planning disorder apraxia. See also chapter 3, which addresses the voice, including good vocal hygiene and diseases and disorders that affect the voice.

Speech Mechanism, Part II: Chewing and Swallowing

> *They told you those are your permanent teeth, but it's a lie.*
> Cynical grandparent to gullible grandchild

When I saw the above joke on the internet, I chuckled over its truth about aging. Unlike what we were told as children in our Tooth Fairy years, our adult teeth are not necessarily permanent. Although eating is not communication, it involves many of the same body parts, so it is an area speech-language pathologists address. Swallowing challenges also occur in adults with neurologically based communication disorders like those addressed in this book.

As our body parts responsible for swallowing age, we may experience changes to how we eat that could affect health and quality of life. Changes in swallowing due to normal aging are called *presbyphagia*. When swallowing becomes a significant challenge, because of a disease or disorder, it's called *dysphagia*. In chapter 4, you will find a clear description of the normal and disordered stages of swallowing. See appendix C for a visual depiction of these body parts, which may help you understand the swallowing process.

McCoy and Desai (2018) explain in their article on presbyphagia and dysphagia that there are several potential challenges in normal aging. These can include tooth loss, poor oral hygiene, decreased saliva, and reduced tongue strength and pressure. There can also be sensory changes, whereby senses of touch, smell, and taste change in ways that affect how we eat and drink. You might, for example, notice food bits across an older person's lips and tongue, or see some food specks fly across the table as a person eats. Adults over 65 years of age may have a slower swallow. They may collect more food in the nooks and crannies of their mouths and throats compared to adults younger than 45 years. Compared to young adults, older adults may also experience more frequent occurrences of food and drink getting into their airways.

This overview of the normal aging swallow, like the other skills addressed in this book, is not exhaustive. It provides an idea of what one might experience. It's wise to stay aware of how well you chew and swallow and consider what ASHA (n.d.) reports as general signs of a disordered swallow. These include coughing or having a wet-sounding voice during or after eating or drinking, increased time or effort for chewing or swallowing, food getting stuck in your mouth, or having food or drink leaking from your lips. Weight loss and trouble breathing following meals can be signs of a swallowing problem too. Another serious sign and potential consequence of poor swallowing is aspiration pneumonia. This can happen when food or liquids enter the lungs instead of the stomach. Again, chapter 4 will have more details and helpful information.

What Are Some Cognitive Changes That Occur with Healthy Aging?

> *As you get older three things happen. First your memory goes,*
> *and then I can't remember the other two.*
> Sir Norman Wisdom, actor and comedian

Language and Cognition

Intellect refers to the mental operations of our brain. Language and cognition are the intellectual abilities that support communication; they are inseparable. Language is a symbol system with rules to combine sounds into words, words into phrases, phrases into paragraphs, and so on. There are even rules for how, when, and why we use language. We then use language through cognitive functions like memory, attention, and retrieval.

As Sir Norman suggests in his quotation above, intellectual functions can decline with age. Healthy decline does not reach abnormal levels, though. We can still communicate and develop new skills, though perhaps not as efficiently or in the same way as in our younger years. The aging brain remains plastic; that is, it can change and learn. See the National Institute of Aging (NIA) website for useful information, such as the article, "How the Aging Brain Affects Thinking" (2017).

An encouraging concept regarding the aging brain is cognitive reserve. This is the brain's ability to function despite decline due to normal aging or diseases, like dementia. Individuals with good cognitive reserve perform better in mental activities than you might expect given their age or disease stage. Reed and colleagues (2011) have found that the amount of education someone has, and how active they keep their brain, can help build reserve. That basically means "use it or lose it." This popular saying applies to our brains as well as to our muscles.

Keep your brain active. Play crossword and other language puzzles, volunteer at a local hospital, learn a new hobby. There are endless possibilities. Considering this promising news, researchers are looking for ways to build cognitive reserve. One area of investigation is the potential benefit for older adults to learn a foreign language. There is evidence that being bilingual, using two (or more) languages, can build this reserve. This notion comes from research, such as that of Bialystok, Craik, and Freedman (2007), showing that bilingual speakers have a later onset of Alzheimer's disease relative to speakers who know only one language.

Now, let's address those infamous "senior moments." The NIA (2017) has a useful website that describes what cognitive behaviors, like memory, organizing, and thinking, look like at various stages of life. They help highlight differences between normal aging and diseases or disorders. I encourage you to visit the site, and the others listed at the end of this chapter. In the meantime, I've summarized their information as follows. Between ages 30 to 40 years, we might not see too many signs of cognitive change, but brain size can decrease gradually. From ages 40 to 50, our ability to remember things in the short term may be less efficient, and complex tasks, like math calculations, may take longer than before. From 50 to 60, multitasking, while still possible, might become more difficult, and learning new skills and information may take more time. From ages 60 to 70, managing and understanding information might take longer, and money management skills may also decline. So make sure you have a good financial adviser well ahead of time! From age 70 and up, we might see the effects of lifestyle, health, and genetic issues arise. We might also expect to see signs of dementia in those with a family history of the disease. You will find more on this topic in chapter 6 of this book.

Let's now talk about the language system we use to express needs, wants, and ideas and to navigate our world. Language is a broad topic, so I'll address some major components. For a more complete picture, consider Burke and Shafto's (2008) chapter on aging language reviewed within different models of cognitive aging. We are likely to see language changes due to cognitive changes. Older adults might be a little slower and less skilled in how they use language relative to when they were younger. Nonetheless, they typically maintain general knowledge about their language and an ability to communicate successfully. Generally, our knowledge of concepts, what we have learned in the past, remains good through the aging process. In fact, older adults' general knowledge can even be better than that of younger adults. Vocabulary knowledge, the number of different words we know, is typically a strength and can grow as we age, though we can see a decline around age 70 and probably even later.

While the vocabulary we know is a relative strength, naming those vocabulary words can be a different story. A well-known change in language skills as we age is the trouble we may have recalling names of people, places, and things. When healthy older folks have word-finding trouble, they typically can recall the general meaning of what they want to say with fair ease. The form of the word is harder. So you might remember how an old classmate wore her hair, but not her name. The name is made up of a string of arbitrary sounds. You might experience the "tip of the tongue" phenomenon whereby you recall some parts of the name. Perhaps, for example, you recall that it starts with an *M* sound or is a two-part name, like Mary Ann or Ann Marie, but the actual name escapes you, at least in that moment.

Language is more than just individual words. We typically communicate in sentences, paragraphs, and conversations. Older adults can understand and produce sentences. They may, however, be less efficient at processing and producing sentences that are longer and more complex compared to younger adults. Older adults may also be less skilled and precise in conversations and storytelling. I am reminded of journalist Robert Quillen's quotation: "As we grow older, our bodies get shorter and our anecdotes longer." As language skills change, we might become less successful at including only the most relevant information in a story we tell, or in ignoring unimportant information. You might have noticed older folks sometimes tell you the same story more than once, forgetting that they already told you.

So how can we tell normal aging from disordered behaviors when they can look very similar? The NIA (2017) reports that signs of the early stages of a cognitive disorder, like Alzheimer's dementia, can include memory loss and misplacing objects in strange places, poor decision making, and having less initiative (e.g., drive, resourcefulness, spirit). The NIA also notes signs of needing more time to complete daily tasks like getting dressed as well as a tendency to get lost or wander about. There also might be changes in personality, such as anxiety and aggression. Language-related symptoms of dementia could include frequently repeating questions and having trouble with naming. On the other hand, it's normal as we age to exercise poor judgment, forget an appointment or what day it is, forget a word, or misplace items once in a while. If these happen frequently, it could be a problem to address with a doctor. For more information on communication and cognitive disorders, see chapters 5 and 6. Appendix D includes an illustration of the brain that may be useful in visualizing the structures of the brain responsible for communication.

What Are Some Social-Emotional Factors to Consider in Healthy Aging?

Age is a question of mind over matter.
If you don't mind, it doesn't matter.
Satchel Paige, American baseball player

We've discussed how communication takes place in a social context, so let's look closer at what older adults face from a social-emotional perspective. Good social-emotional skills can support effective communication, quality of life, and simple safety. *Social* refers to how we interact with others, and *emotional*, our state of mind or feelings. The importance of social-emotional well-being to how we function in every area of our lives is gaining attention and becoming an important component of many school programs. This is nice news for future older adults. Social-emotional skills include self-awareness and management, good decision making, relationship skills, and social awareness. These are skills that help us manage our feelings, set healthy goals, have good relationships, and be responsible. For more information, a helpful resource is the Collaborative for Academic, Social, and Emotional Learning website (www.CASEL.org).

Many older adults experience several considerable social and life changes that could affect emotional health, socialization, and communication. One big life change is retirement. The retiree goes from a structured lifestyle, in which they are productive and essential to an institution, to an environment of less structure. This may lead to the loss of a sense of purpose, value, or direction. Retirees can help keep their minds sharp, bodies strong, and hearts happy by finding an exciting new purpose or stimulating opportunities like volunteering, taking classes at a community center, or joining an athletic club. There is also the potential for isolation with loss of life partners or life in nursing homes.

Changing family dynamics may lead to older adults' children, now adults themselves, taking on the role of caregivers, if not authorities regarding their aging parents. Many times, while well intended, family members and even health care professionals unfairly, and inappropriately, treat an older adult like a child. We unfortunately see this far too often with our patients who have communication disorders, like aphasia and dementia. We saw *John* and *Abby's* children be a bit scolding and forward about telling them what to do in retirement.

There are cases where a sufficiently impaired individual cannot make proper decisions for themselves. We might see this with advanced stages of dementia. Yet in many instances, this is not the case, especially with patients who have aphasia. Individuals with aphasia may have less efficient access to language, but their intellect is largely intact, and they can communicate, though it may need to be in new ways, like writing, gesturing, or using a communication device.

The good news is that research suggests that the emotional abilities of older adults are good despite the challenges of aging. Scheibe and Cartensen (2010) point this out in their article on trends in emotional aging. They note that older adults typically have the motivation and skills to maintain a healthy disposition. Maybe this is what Satchel Paige meant in his quotation at the beginning of this section. Some likely reasons for this may be that a person chooses to be happy, knows that life is short, has a lifetime's experience managing emotions, and uses new strategies to face challenges. Notice *John's* carefree attitude in wearing his wife's very feminine glasses. Cognitive or biological factors may influence how older adults process or react to emotional experiences. We need more research to know more.

If someone is facing a communication disorder, it's often an emotional blow to them and their loved ones. It would be helpful for caregivers to be aware of the potential interaction this may have with normal social-emotional experiences we have with age. Being patient, giving loved ones more time to respond, and using communication strategies covered later in this book could prove helpful. For information particular to social-emotional factors, see chapter 7 on patient and caregiver coping and chapter 8 on using the arts in rehabilitation.

What Are the Important Take-Home Points in This Chapter?

General Aging

- Physical, intellectual, and social-emotional areas of human development influence one another. Many of these skills decline as we age, but these changes are considered normal.

- Normal aging changes can overlap with changes that are disordered. It is important to consult your or your loved one's physician if changes feel significant or interfere with daily living.

Vision and Hearing

- Regular eye and hearing exams are important. Wearing corrective lenses or hearing aids, if needed, is helpful to maintain optimal body, mind, and spirit.

Voice, Articulation, and Fluency

- Older adults continue to have clear speech. Voice quality and breath support may change relatively more with age, though.

Chewing and Swallowing

- Chewing and swallowing can become messier and slower as we age. If someone experiences behaviors like increased coughing, a wet-sounding voice, and food getting stuck, it is important to consult a physician.

Language and Cognition

- We become forgetful and long winded as we get older. If these happen more than occasionally, consult a physician.

Social and Emotional

- Older adults can be emotionally resilient but have potential to become lonely or feel blue. Being optimistic can work wonders.

This chapter summarizes age-related changes in the areas of human development most related to communication. These occur in physical, intellectual, and social-emotional domains, areas that influence one another. Some changes are expected with healthy aging, while others may indicate a disorder. This chapter also introduces topics covered in more detail in later chapters, such as disorders of speech, voice, swallowing, language, and cognition.

If you are reading this book, your loved one may face more than just trying to find their glasses or remembering someone's name, as the chapter title suggests. Your loved one may have significant challenges. Please know that, while you both may need to communicate in a new way, individuals with communication disorders can absolutely communicate, except, perhaps, in the most extreme cases. Many people, even related professionals, are not aware of this or the means to improve communication. We hope this book can help change that, since we, as speech-language pathologists, have the tools and the know-how.

This chapter opens with Okakura's quotation about adjustment to change being the art of life. You and your family may be facing enormous changes with aging, a disease, or an acquired brain injury. Betty Friedan has suggested that age is not lost youth but a new opportunity for strength. While likely difficult, I hope you and your loved one will find opportunity for strength in the challenges you may face. I encourage you also to remember Martin Luther King Jr.'s words, "If you can't fly, run; if you can't run, walk; if you can't walk, crawl; but by all means keep moving." It's our hope that this book will help you do that.

REFERENCES

American Academy of Ophthalmology (AAO). (2015, September 8). *Remember your eyes when it comes to fighting the signs of aging.* https://www.aao.org/newsroom/news-releases/detail/remember-your-eyes-when-it-comes-to-fighting-signs.

American Speech-Language-Hearing Association (ASHA). *Swallowing disorders in adults.* https://www.asha.org/public/speech/swallowing/swallowing-disorders-in-adults/.

Bialystok, E., Craik, F. I. M., & Freedman, M. (2007). Bilingualism as a protection against the onset of symptoms of dementia. *Neuropsychologia,* 45(2), 459–64. https://doi.org/10.1016/j.neuropsychologia.2006.10.009.

Burke, D. M., & Shafto, M. A. (2008). Language and aging. In F. I. M. Craik and T. A. Salthouse (Eds.), *The Handbook of Aging and Cognition* (3rd ed., pp. 373–443). Erlbaum.

Ciorba, A., Bianchini, C., Pelucchi, S., & Pastore, A. (2012). The impact of hearing loss on the quality of life of elderly adults. *Clinical Interventions in Aging, 20*, 159–63. https://doi.org/10.2147/CIA.S26059.

Dentone, P., & Afshari, N. (2019, October 22). *Presbyopia*. American Academy of Ophthalmology. https://eyewiki.org/Presbyopia.

Hooper, C. R., & Cralidis, A. (2009). Normal changes in the speech of older adults: You've still got what it takes; it just takes a little longer! *Perspectives on Gerontology, 14*(2), 47–56. https://doi.org/10.1044/gero14.2.47.

Koehnke, J., Lister, J., & Wambacq, I. (2015). Already gone. *ASHA Leader, 20*(6), 38–42. https://doi.org/10.1044/leader.FTR1.20062015.38.

Lin, F. R., Yaffee, K., Xia, J., Xue, Q., Harris, T. B., Purchase-Helzner, E., Satterfield, S., Anonayon, H. N., Ferrucci, L., & Simonsick, E. M. (2013). Hearing loss and cognitive decline among older adults, *JAMA Internal Medicine, 173*(4), 293–99. https://doi.org/10.1001/jamainternmed.2013.1868.

McCoy, Y. M., & Desai, R. V. (2018). Presbyphagia versus dysphagia: Identifying age-related changes in swallow function. *Perspective of the ASHA Special Interest Groups, 3*(15), 15–21. https://doi.org/10.1044/persp3.SIG15.15.

Mukamal, R. (2015, September 11). *Fighting the signs of aging? Don't forget the eyes.* American Academy of Ophthalmology. https://www.aao.org/eye-health/news/fighting-signs-of-aging-don-t-forget-eyes.

National Eye Institute. National Institutes of Health (2019, June). *Taking Care of Your Vision After 50.* https://www.nei.nih.gov/sites/default/files/2019-06/Taking-Care-Your-Vision-After-50.pdf

National Institute on Aging (NIA). (2017, May 17). *How the aging brain affects thinking.* https://www.nia.nih.gov/health/how-aging-brain-affects-thinking.

National Institute on Deafness and Other Communication Disorders (NIDCD). (2016, March). *Hearing loss and older adults.* https://www.nidcd.nih.gov/sites/default/files/Documents/health/hearing/HearingLossOlderAdults.pdf.

National Institute on Deafness and Other Communication Disorders (NIDCD). (2018, July 17). *Age-related hearing loss.* https://www.nidcd.nih.gov/health/age-related-hearing-loss.

Owsley, C. (2016). Vision and aging. *Annual Review of Vision Science, 2*, 255–71. https://doi.org/10.1146/annurev-vision-111815-114550.

Reed. B. R., Dowling, M., Tomaszewski Farias, S., Sonnen, J., Strauss, M., Schneider, J. A., Bennett, D. A., & Mungas, D. (2011). Cognitive activities during adulthood are more important than education in building reserve. *Journal of the International Neuropsychological Society, 17*(4), 615–24. https://doi.org/10.1017/S1355617711000014.

Rodgers, A. M., & Langa, K. M. (2010). Untreated poor vision: A contributing factor to late-life dementia. *American Journal of Epidemiology, 171*(6), 728–35. https://doi.org/10.1093/aje/kwp453.

Scheibe, S., & Carstensen, L. L. (2010). Emotional aging: Recent findings and future trends. *Journal of Gerontology: Psychological Sciences, 65B*(2), 135–44. https://doi.org/10.1093/geronb/gbp132.

US Census Bureau. (2017, August 3). *Facts for features: Older Americans month, May 2017.* https://www.census.gov/newsroom/facts-for-features/2017/cb17 -ffo8.html.

RESOURCES

American Psychological Association: https://www.apa.org/index.aspx

American Speech-Language and Hearing Association: https://www.asha.org

Collaborative for Academic, Social, and Emotional Learning (CASEL): https://www.CASEL.org.

National Eye Health Education Program (NEHEP): https://nei.nih.gov/nehep

National Health Information Center Clearinghouses: https://www.nidcd.nih .gov/health/clearinghouse

National Institute on Aging: https://www.nia.nih.gov

National Institute on Deafness and Other Communication Disorders (NIDCD): https://www.nidcd.nih.gov

Office of Disease Prevention and Health Promotion (ODPHP): https://health .gov/about-odphp

Psychology Today: https://www.psychologytoday.com/us

US Department of Health and Human Services: https://www.hhs.gov

ABOUT THE AUTHOR

Dr. Teresa Signorelli Pisano is a speech-language pathologist and cognitive scientist. She is a former Visiting Research Scholar in the PhD Program in Speech-Language-Hearing Sciences at the CUNY Graduate Center and clinic director in the Communication Sciences and Disorder Department a Marymount Manhattan College. Dr. Signorelli Pisano's clinical work and research has addressed the bilingual brain across the lifespan. Her latest work examines brain-based changes in healthy aging and second-language acquisition.

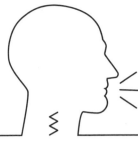

TWO

Communication Is a Two-Way Street

Understanding and Coping with Unclear Speech

Connie K. Porcaro, PhD, CCC-SLP

Mary, who has Parkinson's disease, is having a rough day. She isn't feeling very well, and so far, her medicines have not kicked in to help her be able to move as she would like. It's still early yet, so she is hoping they will make her feel better soon. As she lies in bed, she realizes that what she really needs is a cool drink of water. Her husband, David, is a great caregiver and always wants to give her everything she needs. She licks her dry lips and calls, "David?" hoping he may hear her from the kitchen, where he is emptying the dishwasher. She feels unsteady and doesn't trust getting out of bed and to the kitchen on her own. "David?" she tries again but realizes he can't hear her over the clanking of the dishes. Mary feels helpless and depressed that she needs to rely so much on someone else for such a simple thing.

Tony had a stroke two months ago, and despite attending speech therapy, he still has difficulty speaking in a loud, clear voice. His wife, Suzanne, can usually understand most of what he says. The thing he struggles with the most is the weekly Sunday afternoon conversations he has with his three grandchildren. It has been a family ritual that the grandkids call him after church, and he missed that so much when he was in the

43

hospital. As soon as he got home, he was looking forward to that precious weekly call, but he found that his grandchildren (ages 3, 5, and 8) didn't seem able to understand him over the phone. His daughter tried to interpret what he was saying, but sometimes even she couldn't understand him.

What Are Some Ways That Communication Can Break Down?

Understanding loved ones is critical to happiness, effective relationships, and proper care of aging individuals. If speech is not clear and easily understood, both the speaker and the listener can become frustrated, and the best care may not happen. We think of communication as being the responsibility of the speaker. But what if a speaker has difficulty getting their message across clearly? Other factors can also affect the ability of a person's message to make it to their communication partner. In fact, the listener also shares the responsibility of making sure they understand the message. Another factor that affects whether the message gets through is the communication environment, which involves factors surrounding the individuals.

In the first case presented above, *Mary* is the speaker, or the person who is attempting to get a message to her husband, *David*. We can define their communication environment as the house they live in. Remember, in the case above, *Mary* is in the bedroom, and *David* is in the kitchen, so they have a large shared communication environment because they are not in the same room. Because she has Parkinson's disease, *Mary's* message will probably be harder to understand, even under the best conditions. People with Parkinson's disease generally have very slow, small movements in their entire body. This often results in speech being very soft and hard to understand. Beyond that, the communication environment is providing a tremendous challenge here. *David* is in another room and has environmental distractions from the noise of the dishes as he puts them away.

The second case involves a speaker, *Tony*, who is struggling to be understood over the phone. The listeners include his daughter and his grandchildren. Talking on the phone can be a challenging communication environment because of a poor connection and lack of a typical face-to-face experience. As listeners, we use information such as lip movements to help us understand certain words and sounds. But on the phone, *Tony* can't see his granddaughter's face if she makes a puzzled expression when she doesn't understand him. *Tony*'s speech difficulties as a result of his stroke have made this situation more difficult.

The rest of this chapter addresses why these types of communication breakdowns can occur between loved ones and their caregivers. You will learn strategies to help improve communication. Both the speaker and the communication partner / listener can use these strategies to improve the communication environment. So even though we usually think about the speaker as being primarily responsible for communication, it's important to realize it's a two-way street. The listener should also be active in the process and can help create a better communication environment.

Why Do People with Neurological Diseases or Injuries Have Difficulty Speaking Clearly?

When an acquired brain injury or a degenerative disease is the reason that a person has difficulty being understood, a medical diagnosis will likely come from a neurologist. Medical diagnoses that relate to speech difficulties might include a stroke, Parkinson's disease, multiple sclerosis, or amyotrophic lateral sclerosis (Lou Gehrig's disease). Two main speech issues can occur in adults with neurological conditions: dysarthria and apraxia of speech, which are also known as *motor speech disorders*. These speech disorders are different from problems with language, typically called *aphasia* (see chapter 5). Dysarthria occurs when there is weakness or incoordination in the parts of the body involved in speech. These include the respiratory, or breathing, system (lungs and airways); the phonatory, or voicing, system (larynx or voice box); and the speech (articulation) system, which helps move our mouth and tongue in forming sounds, words, and sentences. In some cases, air may excessively escape through the nose instead of the mouth, making the person sound "nasally." Appendix A shows the structures that help us produce speech. Someone who has had a stroke, like *Tony*, might have unclear speech because of weakness in the lips and tongue. Someone who has Parkinson's disease might have very quiet speech because of weak muscles in the lungs and voice box. Apraxia of speech occurs when a person's brain does not properly execute the plan to tell the muscles how to make speech sounds. In either disorder, the speech may not be understood if it is not clear or loud enough. The impact of either speech disorder is that caregivers may have great difficulty understanding the needs and thoughts of their loved ones.

Any acquired injury or degenerative disease that affects how the brain tells our muscles to move will often keep a person from being able to speak clearly. Different diseases or injuries may impair the body in different ways. For more information on specific acquired brain injuries or degenerative diseases, please see the list of resources at the end of this chapter.

On the topic of getting a clear message across, it's important to review how illness can affect how we talk. First, some people will have very mild speech issues, while others may have severe difficulties communicating. This can also change within a person as a disease (like Parkinson's disease or amyotrophic lateral sclerosis) progresses or possibly improves with medication or treatment. So there can be decline or improvement over time. Sometimes loved ones who have had a stroke will experience *spontaneous recovery*. This is a time, usually soon after the stroke, when the brain and nerves are healing, and speech may improve on its own.

How Do We Make Sounds, Words, and Sentences into Something a Listener Understands?

When we speak, we take a breath into our lungs and then exhale, or blow it out. During exhalation, the air moves through our trachea (windpipe) and vibrates two small bands of muscle tissue called the vocal folds (or vocal cords). Vibrations of the vocal folds create our voice. Our voice is then directed through our nose and mouth to produce a distinctive sound. The sound gets formed further by the way we move our lips, tongue, and jaw. Take a breath and try making a *B* sound. When you make that sound, you trap air in your mouth by closing your lips tightly and then letting that sound burst out. Now try making an *F* sound. This time, you are forcing a stream of air to move through your teeth, which are touching your lower lip. We create distinct speech sounds by moving different parts of our mouth, such as our lips and tongue.

Now, let's review how breakdowns in clear communication can arise from difficulties related to moving certain parts of the body. When we are speaking, we can control the air as it leaves our lungs to help us get to the end of a sentence. Speakers who have neurological issues may not have this control of their exhaled air. If a person has reduced respiration, or ability to control the air they are breathing, they may get winded and run out of air in the middle of words or sentences. This person may also take breaths at unexpected times when they are speaking. Sometimes, people with neurological issues cannot use the air to create a voice through vocal fold vibrations.

When this happens, we may hear their voice break or just stop working when they are speaking. Sometimes, their voice will be very quiet. Their voice could also sound breathy or tense while they are speaking, depending on the type of acquired brain injury or degenerative disease they have.

If an acquired brain injury or degenerative disease does not allow normal movement of the lips, tongue, or jaw, your loved one may be difficult to understand. You may hear slurred, unclear speech. One other problem that can also affect our ability to understand a speaker's message is how nasally their voice sounds. If certain structures are not working correctly, a person's voice can sound too nasally or have very little nasal sound (the way we sound when we have a stuffy nose). In some cases, this can cause a person to be difficult to understand.

How Might Speech-Language Pathologists Help Your Loved One Improve Communication?

If your loved one is having difficulty communicating, there is someone who can help. Please reach out to a speech-language pathologist, or SLP. Your loved one's general physician or neurologist will help you find an SLP. This person has the training and experience in working with breakdowns in communication. The SLP will complete an evaluation to know exactly what problems are affecting your loved one's ability to speak. Many times, SLPs have therapy techniques that can be helpful. For example, if a person has difficulty using the air from their lungs appropriately, SLPs can work on improving their posture. Another great strategy might include teaching the person to take a larger breath and to control the breath as it leaves the lungs. We can improve breath control, but it can require hours of practice. If a person's voice is too soft, which often happens with Parkinson's disease or other disorders, SLPs can use programs that help the person develop a stronger and louder voice. These programs include Lee Silverman Voice Treatment (LSVT) and SPEAK OUT! / LOUD Crowd (see the resources at the end of this chapter). SLPs can also practice strategies to help make a person's speech clearer by instruction and practice on particular speech sounds. An SLP may also ask the person to practice using a slower rate of speech. Overall, if your loved one is difficult to understand, an SLP is the best person to see.

In more severe situations, the SLP may determine that a device would be helpful to assist a person in making their needs and wants understood. This might be in the form of a board that the person can point to that has pictures of basic words (e.g., bed, water, toilet). It could also be a high-tech device that can speak for the person. There are also many options in between, but an SLP is a great resource to help you and your loved one find the best way to communicate. We call these augmentative/alternative communication, or AAC, devices. Naturally, most people would rather keep communicating by speaking. Sometimes, a person's speech cannot be understood if a disease that is affecting the brain progresses to a serious point. If your loved one is considering the use of an AAC device, it is important to start early. This allows the SLP to communicate easily with them while selecting and training with a device. Also, some devices can be programmed with a person's actual voice (as opposed to a more robotic option). While the person can still be understood, their voice can be "banked" to be used in the device. Voice banking allows for recording a person's voice, which can then be programmed into an AAC device. Some options for voice banking include the ModelTalker, CereVoice Me, MyVocaliD, and My Own Voice (see resources at the end of this chapter). These types of devices do not need to be used at all times. Sometimes, a person can use their own voice for some situations, while in others, they might need to use an AAC device. Someone dealing with amyotrophic lateral sclerosis (ALS) might eventually need an AAC device as their ability to communicate lessens. Regular visits to the SLP will keep this person on track for knowing how to best communicate as their disease progresses. Please talk with an SLP to help you make this important decision with your loved one.

What Are Some Strategies That Speakers Can Use to Be Better Understood?

Someone who is dealing with an acquired brain injury or a degenerative disease may be prevented from making the movements required for speech that is understandable to others. Individuals who are not understood will find it frustrating if they cannot make their needs, wants, and ideas known to caregivers or others in their life. A person may find it embarrassing to rely on someone else to communicate for them. If communicating effectively is an issue, it is important to see an SLP. The SLP can begin an evaluation to determine exactly what might be most useful in improving a person's ability to communicate. They can also provide therapy to help instruct individuals in the best ways to be understood. Most people can easily use the suggestions in the next few sections to improve the clarity of their speech.

Speaker Strategies

Let's go back to the first story from the beginning of this chapter. There are some fixable problems in the story of Mary trying to communicate with her husband, David. First, it is important for David to know that Mary is attempting to speak to him. The best way to communicate is face to face, so getting in the same room is critical. Since Mary is having difficulty moving, she and David should set up a system that enables her to get his attention from a distance. A whistle or bell that Mary can use easily would be a good signal to David that she needs to speak with him. So a good starting point is for a person to get the attention of their communication partner before they start talking. Even if they are in the same room, the potential listener may not be fully attentive without a signal. Maintaining eye contact while speaking is also helpful. For example, in the earlier scenario, even if *Mary* and *David* had both been in the kitchen, the clanking noise of the dishes as *David* was cleaning up may have made it difficult for her to get his attention. Many years of research have taught us that seeing a person's mouth and face move during speech can provide useful clues, even when speakers do not have any communication problems. We may often rely on lip reading if there is loud background noise or if the speaker is close but still hard to understand. The visual movements of speech are also useful when speakers have speech that is hard to understand, as can happen with Parkinson's disease (Keintz, Bunton, & Hoit, 2007) or stroke. The same advice applies to *Tony*'s dilemma in trying to communicate with his family over the phone. Again, in this situation, the listener misses out on useful and important visual clues.

The speaker should start by introducing the topic, so they provide the communication partner with some context for what will be discussed. After *Mary* gets *David* into the room and he can see her face, she can start with an easy message like "I'm thirsty." A supportive caregiver like *David* may also start the conversation by asking, "What can I do to help you?" Either way, these statements will introduce the topic and will help the listener predict what the speaker might say next. If you think about it, this is just part of a normal conversation. We often start speaking with someone by introducing a topic, for example, "Let me tell you what happened yesterday." This is a good way to set the listener up to know where you want the conversation to go next. Or, if we are changing a topic, it's especially important to be sure that our listener changes topics with us. Again, most of us communicate in that way. For instance, if I am talking to someone about their day, but I want to be sure to tell them about the play I saw, I may say, "Oh, I wanted to tell you about *Hamilton*, the play I just saw." This alerts the listener that I am switching to a new topic. This information is even more important for speakers who have trouble being understood. The listener will have a much easier time understanding the message if they have a good idea of the topic being discussed. In the second story that began this chapter, *Tony* had difficulty being understood by his daughter and grandchildren. He could try introducing the topic, such as starting with "I wanted to tell you about my fishing trip." This way, they know keywords to listen for to help them understand him.

This paragraph contains strategies you can share with your loved one if they are having trouble being understood. Teach them to try to make their messages easily understood. Use complete but simple sentences. Don't leave out important words if they will help the listener understand the message. Use predictable wording; for instance, "Bill wants to swim" is easier to understand than "Swimming is what Bill wants to do." If you run out of breath, and your voice quits working, your listener may miss important words. Take breaths as needed to get all words across clearly. Sometimes, your loved one may need to take a quick breath between each word or every couple of words. That is better than running out of air and having the listener miss important words in the message. Here's an example of how *Mary* can get her message across to *David* (imagine that the slash lines are where *Mary* takes her breaths). "/I'm/ thirsty/." *Mary* might need two breaths, even for that brief message. Taking breaths between words and not in the middle of a word is also a good idea. If *Mary* said, "/I/ /am/ /wait/ /ing/ f/or/ a/ dr/ink/," the breaths she is taking are breaking up the short words. So, the right balance here is to take enough breaths to get words out, but not so many that the words or syllables are broken down by the breaths. This will vary from person to person and may change through a loved one's disease process or even just throughout the day. Fatigue will be a factor in this, so if a person is more tired than usual, they may need to take it slow and take more breaths. Another useful strategy is to overenunciate words. Tell your loved one to imagine they are speaking to someone who is hard of hearing and they need to speak slowly and clearly. They should keep in mind that people whom they talk to frequently will probably understand them better than anyone else. If they are communicating with someone new, they may need to use more effort and work extra hard to get the message across.

A speaker and their communication partner should make a plan for communication breakdowns. Some speakers may feel comfortable if a listener interrupts them to ask questions or clarify. Others may want to get the complete sentence or thought out before they get this feedback. There should also be a plan for how the listener will let the speaker know they don't understand. As a speaker, do you want the listener to guess at what you are saying and try to finish your sentence? Some people would prefer this, while others would not find it helpful. Communicating about how to best communicate is always a good idea. As speakers, you should be checking with your communication partners to see if they understand. You can look for signs of understanding or confusion. If *Mary* tells *David* that she is thirsty, and he brings her a sandwich, she can be sure the message didn't get to him. If a listener is not getting the message, the speaker will need to consider some "repair" strategies. We use these every day when someone can't understand what we say. If someone says, "What?" our usual strategy is to repeat what we said. Speakers can also attempt to use more effort to speak louder and overenunciate a misunderstood message.

It's critical for speakers who may have problems getting their message across verbally to use all other available options for getting out their needs, wants, and ideas. If *David* does not understand when *Mary* tells him she is thirsty, she has other options. The most obvious is probably to put her hand to her mouth and use the universal sign for drink. Gesturing can be beneficial and can even be used as a supplement when the person is speaking (Hustad & Weismer, 2007). If a spoken message isn't understood, we have other options for communication. We can express messages in many ways. If a listener is having a hard time understanding a single word, spelling out the letters may be helpful. Pointing to what we need can also be a useful way to communicate. If a person is ordering in a restaurant, is there a picture on the menu of the item they would like? If so, rather than speaking for your loved one, ask them to point. If possible, a person may use written communication to help get a message across. Drawing a picture or writing a word or letters may help a listener understand when speech isn't clear. Your loved one could also practice ordering specific items before you head to the restaurant, so that they feel comfortable ordering their meal themselves. Making a facial expression, such as a big smile, is a useful way of expressing how we feel about something. For tech savvy individuals, typing on a keyboard or texting on a phone might be helpful options. A speaker who has difficulty getting their message across should always have a back-up plan for when someone can't understand what they need. Back to *Mary* and *David* for a minute. If *David* is not understanding *Mary's* spoken or gestured message, she could point to a glass of water or her mouth or write a message if needed.

An SLP can also help with some communication options that involve technology. If volume is a problem, a person could use a small portable voice amplifier. Teachers and coaches often use small, fairly inexpensive voice amplifiers so that they can be louder while not overusing their voice by having to shout. Your loved one may only need to rely on this device on a bad day, when fatigue is an issue. A person may need to have an important conversation or give a speech, and the amplifier may be useful. SLPs can also assist with different AAC devices. One option for this, which involves low-level technology, is an alphabet board. (See the example alphabet board in appendix B). A person can use an alphabet board by pointing to the first letter of each word in a sentence. This helps the communication process in two ways. First, the listener is now being provided with the first letter of each word. Also, using an alphabet board slows down the speaker's rate, which helps listeners understand better. In the list of strategies described above, there is likely something that can maximize communication for most people dealing with an acquired brain injury or a degenerative disease. It's also acceptable, however, for people to just need down time, or quiet time when they aren't expected to communicate. Be sure your loved one knows that you understand there will be days or times when they are just tired and don't need to talk as much.

What Are Some Strategies that Communication Partners Can Use to Understand Better?

The communication partner, or listener, also has responsibilities in making sure that their loved one's message is getting through. Even though a long list of speaker strategies was just provided, remember that the speaker in this situation has an acquired brain injury or a degenerative disease that is affecting their ability to communicate. There may be some issues that the speaker cannot overcome. This is where the listener comes in.

Listener Strategies

There are also strategies you can take to be an active partner and listener in an exchange of information. First, give all your attention to the speaker and focus on understanding their message. In our story about *Tony* trying to talk to his grandchildren on the phone, his daughter is the listener go-between, or translator, in this situation. *Tony's* grandchildren may need guidance from her to keep them from being distracted while speaking with him on the phone. You can help focus your attention by being in the same room as the speaker and maintaining eye contact. You really will get more information from your loved one if you can see their face while they speak. To focus completely, you will need to reduce distractions in the room and try not to multitask. Let your loved one know that their message is the most important task at that moment. Provide feedback and encouragement. It's important that you know the speaker strategies in the previous section of this chapter so you can encourage the speaker to use as many strategies as needed for effective communication. As a caregiver, you can also learn to be successful at predicting the needs of your loved one. In our earlier scenario, *David* may have lived with *Mary* long enough to know that she will have movement difficulty and a dry mouth first thing in the morning. He can make sure he is nearby if she needs help.

Make a plan with your communication partner about how to enhance your understanding. Talk to your loved one about whether they want you to interrupt immediately when you don't understand or to ask questions afterward. Signal to the speaker if you don't understand something they have said. Again, this may be something the speaker wants you to do immediately or after they have finished. But don't just answer "yes" to what you don't understand. It is very frustrating to have someone pretend they understand when they clearly did not. Let your loved one know if you did not understand their message. One of the least helpful things you can ask is simply "What?" It is better to be specific about what information you are missing. Let your communication partner know exactly what you didn't understand. For example, *David* may say to *Mary*, "I know you want something to drink, but do you want water or juice?" Now, *Mary* knows *David* gets the key point of her message (she's thirsty), and she can focus the next word or sentence on exactly what she wants to drink. Make a backup plan with the speaker about how to handle a communication breakdown and encourage them to use the strategies listed above, such as gesturing or writing. Be the greatest listener you can be and use all your senses for that job. If you are hard of hearing, see an audiologist or ENT (ear, nose, and throat specialist) to see if hearing aids will be helpful. If you wear glasses, keep them on so you can see the movements of your loved one's mouth and face during communication. Remember, when dealing with someone who is struggling to communicate, a listener can share much of the responsibility for the message getting through. Knowing what your loved one wants, needs, and how they feel is critical to you being an effective partner and caregiver.

What Are Some Ways to Change the Environment to Improve Communication?

Besides using the previously discussed speaker and listener strategies, we can also change the communication environment to be sure all messages are getting through. Since there are already strikes against a speaker who is having difficulty communicating, we want to optimize the environment to help them out as much as possible. There are some simple strategies you can use to create a great communication environment.

Communication Environment Strategies

Reduce, or better yet eliminate, background noise. There are many background noises that we grow accustomed to being around and may just ignore. Make the setting for conversation as quiet as possible. Don't just turn the volume on the TV or radio down; turn it off completely or mute it. Fans or some household appliances (for example, dishwasher or washing machine) can also provide a great deal of distracting background noise. Hold conversations away from these noises whenever possible. Sometimes your loved one will try to communicate in an environment where you can't control the noise. If you find yourself in a noisy place like a restaurant, try to be away from the sources of noise. Ask for a quieter table and sit away from others when possible. If there is noise that you cannot control (for example, traffic or other people), then you need to rely more heavily on the previously described speaker and listener strategies to overcome that noisy, distracting background. Since we know that seeing the speaker's mouth will help us as listeners, be sure you are face to face and avoid having a bright light or sunlight right behind the speaker, which makes it hard to see their mouth movements. You can plan important conversations for a time and place when you know communication strategies can be used. Remember that your loved one may have times of the day when they feel less fatigue and when the effects of medication are helping them the most. This is a time to make phone calls to family members or have important talks. Using Skype, Zoom, Facebook Messenger, or FaceTime may be helpful in speaking with distant relatives or friends, so they can see your loved one as they speak. These options would be excellent ideas to help *Tony* have his weekly communication with his grandchildren. *Mary* and *David* had some environmental issues working against them. Not being in the same room was a huge disadvantage to *Mary* being able to let *David* know she was feeling fatigued and thirsty. You can't possibly always be in the room with your loved one. So you need to make a plan for how they can get your attention from a distance when needed. *Mary* and *David* need to find a system that works, perhaps a bell she can ring to let him know she needs him. Wireless doorbells often work well, and the noise carries across the house with a simple button push. Given *Mary*'s weakened state, it might be hard for her to speak clearly, so having him in the room, looking at her face, and completely focused on understanding her message will be the best way to communicate.

What Are the Consequences of Not Being Understood?

Effective communication with other people is a skill that many people experience in their first year of life. To lose that ability is a difficult consequence that often comes with disease or injury that affects the brain. We take communication for granted until it is compromised. When someone is ill and depends on others for their care, feeding, and grooming, they may have many messages they need to share. A person with neurological issues will experience many changes and difficulties, such as loss of movement and independence. In addition to that, communication with loved ones, physicians, and caregivers can be compromised. This is particularly frustrating when your loved one remains cognitively sharp. Speakers with these issues may become frustrated and find it easier to simply withdraw from interaction with others. Since it is more challenging to take part in former life activities, the person may stop interacting with others as much as they would have previously. Our quality of life depends so much on feeling well, which requires good communication with physicians and caregivers. But quality of life also depends highly on social interactions. Please use as many of the strategies in this chapter as you can to help yourself and your loved one. Seeing an SLP will also lead to a useful management plan that could be set up to meet a person's individual needs.

What Are the Important Take-Home Points in This Chapter?

- Our ability to produce understandable speech involves the coordination of many parts of our body working together, including the lungs, vocal cords, lips, and tongue.

- Dysarthria and apraxia are speech disorders that can affect a person's ability to be understood, due to an acquired brain injury or a degenerative disease, such as Parkinson's disease.

- Use the best means of communication that works, whether that involves speech, writing, gestures, or a combination of these.

- Remember that speech therapy can improve someone's ability to communicate, so seek out a speech-language pathologist for an evaluation and management plan when communication is a challenge.

- Changing the communication environment, such as turning off background noise, can improve a listener's ability to understand a speaker.

- Both the speaker and listener can change how they are interacting to improve communication.

Communication between caregivers and loved ones is a critical component to successful management of acquired brain injuries or degenerative diseases. While there may be many challenges to effective communication in this situation, multiple strategies can improve the ability of loved ones to express their wants, needs, and ideas to caregivers. These strategies can include changes to the loved one's behaviors, the caregiver's behaviors, and the environment in which they are communicating. Having a plan for effective communication can decrease frustration and improve the quality of their lives. Keep that "two-way street" an open highway for meaningful communication.

REFERENCES

Hustad, K. C. & Weismer, G. (2007). A continuum of interventions for individuals with dysarthria: Compensatory and rehabilitative treatment approaches. In G. Weismer (Ed.), *Motor Speech Disorders: Essays for Ray Kent* (pp. 261–303). Plural.

Keintz, C. K., Bunton, K., & Hoit, J. D. (2007). Influence of visual information on the intelligibility of dysarthric speech. *American Journal of Speech-Language Pathology, 6*, 222–34.

RESOURCES

American Speech-Language-Hearing Association: https://www.asha.org
   Apraxia of Speech in Adults: https://www.asha.org/public/speech/disorders/Apraxia-of-Speech-in-Adults/
   Augmentative and Alternative Communication (AAC): https://www.asha.org/public/speech/disorders/AAC/
   Dysarthria: https://www.asha.org/public/speech/disorders/dysarthria/
Lee Silverman Voice Treatment (LSVT): https://www.lsvtglobal.com/
Parkinson Voice Project: https://www.parkinsonvoiceproject.org
   SPEAK OUT!/LOUD Crowd Programs: https://www.parkinsonvoiceproject.org/SPEAKOUT
Stroke Association: https://www.stroke.org.uk
   Life after Stroke: Helping Someone with Communication Problems: https://www.stroke.org.uk/sites/default/files/helping_someone_with_communication_problems.pdf
Voice-Banking Options
   ModelTalker: https://www.modeltalker.org
   CereVoice Me: https://www.cereproc.com/en/cerevoice-me
   MyVocaliD: https://vocalid.ai/myvocalid/
   Acapela Group, Voice Banking: https://acapela-group.com/voices/voice-banking/

ABOUT THE AUTHOR

Dr. Connie Porcaro is an Associate Professor in the Department of Communication Sciences and Disorders at Florida Atlantic University (FAU). She received her BA in Communication Sciences and Disorders from the University of South Dakota, her MA in Speech Pathology from the University of Northern Colorado, and her PhD in Speech and Hearing Sciences from the University of Arizona. Dr. Porcaro instructs courses at FAU covering voice, speech, and swallowing disorders in adults. She lectures annually for the FAU Charles E. Schmidt College of Medicine on the topics of adult neurogenic communication disorders.

Dr. Porcaro is certified by the American Speech-Language-Hearing Association and has worked as a speech-language pathologist for more than twenty-five years with clients of all ages. Her primary area of research has focused on intelligibility in patients with speech and voice disorders and how speakers can improve communication with their listeners. She has published research articles in top journals, including the *American Journal of Speech-Language Pathology* and the *International Journal of Speech-Language Pathology*. Dr. Porcaro is a frequent presenter at the Annual Convention of the American Speech-Language-Hearing Association and often presents for state association conventions as an invited speaker. She is an active member of the Leadership Team Professional Development Subcommittee for the American Speech-Language-Hearing Association Special Interest Group on Neurophysiology and Neurogenic Speech and Language Disorders. She has received grant funding from the FAU Healthy Aging Research Initiative to investigate voice and swallowing changes in healthy elderly participants. Dr. Porcaro has received grant funding from the Parkinson Voice Project to facilitate training for graduate students who provide free speech therapy for individuals with Parkinson's disease.

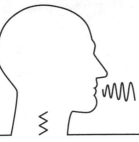

THREE

An Owner's Guide to a Healthy Voice

Connie K. Porcaro, PhD, CCC-SLP

Tuesday at noon: "I need to blah blah blah"—Joyce heard her husband's words, but his voice was so quiet toward the end that she could not make out what he needed. "What?" she yelled from the kitchen. She felt a slight bit of pain in her throat as she yelled. Zach had the television turned up very loud, so she had to really strain for him to hear her from the other room. After hearing another muffled attempt, she left dinner on the stove and went to him. "I need to eat soon so I can take my medicine," Zach said. Joyce had noticed for months that his voice wasn't nearly as loud as it used to be. And definitely not since his doctor had diagnosed him with Parkinson's disease. His doctor had mentioned that his voice would become quieter as the disease progressed. But why was her voice becoming a problem? Surely she didn't have Parkinson's disease as well?

Thursday morning: Joyce took Zach to see the speech-language pathologist (SLP). She felt shaky from drinking three cups of coffee that morning, just to stay with it. Her own voice came out more as a croak as she spoke to the receptionist about Zach's voice issues. In a few minutes, they sat down with Kathy, the SLP, who took notes and asked questions related to Zach's voice. Joyce did most of the talking, assuming it would be easier for Kathy to understand her, but her voice felt tired and slightly painful when she talked. If only she'd had a cigarette; that would have taken the edge off. Her last one had been several hours ago.

Three weeks later: Communication between Joyce and Zach was much better since they had both learned how to take care of their voices. The SLP, Kathy, realized right away that Joyce was struggling with her voice. Kathy taught Joyce that some of her voice issues were because of her age, and the way she was overusing her voice caused other issues. Some minor changes helped with the way her voice sounded and with the feeling of fatigue she was having when she spoke. She was working on giving up smoking completely (one day at a time) and was down to one cup of coffee and many more cups of water in a day. Also, Kathy had taught her that she had to be in the room with Zach, even looking right at his mouth so she could understand him. Zach's voice was also somewhat louder as well. He had enrolled in speech therapy sessions with Kathy to learn techniques to help use his breath support to make his voice louder. While Joyce and Zach knew they had a tough road ahead of them, they suspected the road would be easier if they could communicate more effectively and begin taking ownership of their voices.

This chapter covers the topic of voice disorders. The way we use our voices can cause some voice disorders, as with *Joyce* in the story above. We can also experience voice problems related to disease, injury, or even just the normal aging process.

How Does Your Voice Work?

Parts of your body provide air and filters to help produce your voice. The illustration in appendix A shows you these structures. The sound of your voice comes from air moving from the lungs through your larynx, or voice box. The larynx sits directly on top of the trachea, or windpipe. The larynx has two bands of smooth muscle tissue, or vocal cords, which vibrate when air from your lungs moves through them. The sound produced by those vibrations is your voice. Sounds then move through your throat, nose, and mouth. These structures help shape the sound into words and sentences. The quality of your voice can involve its pitch, loudness, and tone. The size and shape of the vocal cords and the cavities the sound moves through, such as the mouth, nose, and throat, can affect how your voice sounds. This is why people have voices that sound different from each other. You can probably think of someone you know or someone famous who has a distinctive voice. The actor James Earl Jones has a deep, resonant voice that most people find pleasant. The actress Fran Drescher's voice sounds nasally, which is why we remember her. These two individuals have different vocal cord sizes, and they direct the airflow to different areas to create distinct sounding voices.

What Is a Voice Disorder?

A person's voice is an important window into their personality, behavior, and even health. You can recognize many people without seeing them just by hearing their voice. Like fingerprints, voices are unique. You can also recognize if a person you are close to is ill, tired, or sad just by the way their voice sounds. People can develop voice disorders anytime during their life, sometimes because of how they use their voice, and sometimes related to how their body is functioning. A voice disorder occurs when a person has difficulty in work, school, or social settings as a result of the way their voice sounds. People rely heavily on their voices in their everyday lives but give little thought to what they need to do to maintain a healthy voice. This is even more important in an aging population, among whom minor changes in the voice are common. Weakness of muscles and reduced elasticity can cause a softer, more breathy voice in even healthy individuals as they age. This chapter focuses on the primary ways to keep your voice in its best condition. Age-related voice changes are presented early in the chapter, along with good habits you can use to take care of your voice. Later in the chapter, I discuss the impact of acquired brain injuries and degenerative diseases on a person's voice.

How Do I Know if I Have a Voice Disorder?

Any of the following may be important signs of a voice disorder:

- Changes in your voice, including hoarse, breathy, or raspy quality
- Changes in the pitch (high or low tones) of your voice
- Speaking with reduced or softer volume
- Feeling of achiness, fatigue, or strain in the throat or neck when speaking
- More effort required to speak
- Frequent coughing or throat clearing

If you or a loved one has any of the signs above, consult a doctor to determine the underlying cause. A doctor who specializes in diseases and disorders of the ears, nose, and throat is an ENT doctor, or otolaryngologist. This person may be the best doctor to diagnose voice difficulties. With voice disorders that result from an acquired brain injury or degenerative disease, your loved one will probably see a neurologist. A doctor may refer you and your loved one to a speech-language pathologist (SLP) to help you both learn better ways to use your voices to reduce or eliminate any issues.

Why Do People Develop Voice Disorders?

People can develop voice problems at any time in their life. Medical issues may be related to the cause of some voice disorders. For example, some people develop an upper respiratory infection and then don't really take it easy on their voice. Hard voice use can irritate the delicate tissues of the vocal cords when there is postnasal drip and coughing. This constant irritation can cause the vocal cords to vibrate differently, resulting in a quiet, hoarse voice. Another example of a medical issue that can cause a voice disorder is when there is inflammation caused by acid reflux. This occurs when acids from the stomach that are naturally present to help us digest food move back up through our body toward the chest and neck. This acid can cause the feeling of heartburn, and the acid can wash up as high as our vocal cords, which can damage them. If the acid stays down in the esophagus (the tube food moves through), we call this gastroesophageal reflux disease (GERD). If the acid reflux moves up toward the level of the vocal cords, it is called laryngopharyngeal reflux disease (LPR). While some people feel heartburn and pain, others who have GERD or LPR do not feel any pain but may have a frequent cough. Treatment for reflux disease is often successful with medication but also involves changing behaviors to help alleviate the production and movement of acid. If your doctor diagnoses you or your loved one with GERD or LPR, it is critical to take medications as prescribed and to change behaviors as directed. More serious medical conditions can also be related to voice disorders, including laryngeal cancer and degenerative brain diseases. Signs of these types of disorders would be gradual or rapid voice changes, including a tremor or quiver in the voice, hoarseness lasting more than two weeks, breathy or weak-sounding voice, and pain during speech or when swallowing. Seeking medical help is the first step in determining the cause of a voice problem. Voice issues specific to acquired brain injuries and degenerative diseases are described in more detail later in this chapter.

Some people develop voice disorders because of the way they use their voice. Misuse or overuse of the voice can cause strain and stress on the tissues that help us produce a healthy voice. Jobs that involve constant talking in a noisy environment (teaching, coaching, or telemarketing) may contribute to poor vocal behaviors. Other

times, vocal abuse occurs related to our habits or activities and interests. Some individuals might have a job where they use their voice
often and then sing in the church choir or sing karaoke for fun. Other
people may become loudly involved in sporting events, as a participant, coach, or fan, and may yell and scream in response to their
excitement. An actual growth on the vocal cords may appear, similar
to a blister or lesion, after only one episode of heavy voice use. Or
these episodes can build over time and lead to a more tough growth,
like a callus, on the vocal cords. These growths can alter the way a person's voice sounds, resulting in a breathy, low-pitched, weak-sounding voice. Changing the way we use our voice can improve and sometimes cure these types of voice disorders, which I discuss in a later
section of this chapter.

We now know that many people experience age-related changes
in their voice quality (Boone et al., 2014). We call this condition *pres-*
byphonia. The term *presby* means age related and *phonia* relates to
the voice. So, if you have noticed that your voice does not sound the
same as it did when you were younger, that is probably related to
the effects of the aging process on the muscles and tissues that produce your voice. One common change that we might notice in an
aging voice is a difference in the resonance or tone. A voice that previously sounded rich and resonant may become thinner or weaker
sounding. This occurs when the muscles that move the vocal cords
do not vibrate as effectively as they used to, so your voice doesn't
sound as strong as it did when you were younger. Also, changes in
the size and movements of our lungs occur as we age, further affecting the strength and loudness of our voices (Linville, 2001). Some
people experience a rougher, scratchy-sounding voice as they grow
older. This also occurs as a result of changes in the vocal cords and
the muscles that move them. Untreated GERD or smoking can also
cause a rough-sounding voice. We all recognize a smoker's voice when
we hear one. Many people with presbyphonia, or age-related voice

changes, report that their voice isn't as loud as it once was. Many elderly people exhibit breathing difficulties as they age. Loudness of the voice will be reduced if there is any kind of reduction in how effectively the respiratory system works. Aging individuals may lack the proper breath support to maintain the vocal loudness and force that they formerly used. Researchers who have studied voice changes during the aging process consistently note that our pitch changes as we grow older (Basaraba, 2020). Pitch is how high or low your voice sounds. There may be muscle atrophy, which occurs as the muscles waste away and become smaller. If this occurs, the vocal cords may not work as they used to, which results in a woman's pitch dropping slightly over time (getting lower) and a man's pitch rising (getting higher). Hormonal changes before, during, or after menopause can also cause pitch changes in women. Another common complaint in those with age-related voice problems is vocal fatigue. The muscles and structures that produce your voice can fatigue and fade in their strength as the day goes on. Vocal use will be a big factor here. If you use your voice hard or talk for long periods during the day, you may find that your voice (neck and throat) feels tired and strained later at night.

What Can You Do to Prevent or Improve Voice Disorders?

The first thing to do if you or your loved one experiences voice issues is to seek medical attention. Please be sure to see a doctor if you hear or feel any of the signs mentioned earlier in this chapter. But, to take the best care of your own voice or your loved one's, you should incorporate general principles of vocal hygiene—behaviors and strategies that can prevent and even improve existing voice disorders. Everyone, at any age, can have their best-sounding voice by protecting their "instrument" (the vocal cords). These strategies may apply to you, the caregiver, or to your loved one. You may find that both of you use them.

Food and Drinks

Some suggestions in this section relate to GERD to ease those symptoms, but overall, the ideas here will support a healthy and functional voice for anyone. It's important to keep hydrated by drinking at least eight cups (64 oz) of water a day. This level of water intake will help keep mucus that forms in the throat thin, which should help eliminate coughing and throat clearing (which are both abusive behaviors for the voice). A healthy amount of water intake will also keep the structures that produce the voice hydrated, which is needed for a healthy voice. It's a good idea to check with your doctor to see what amount of water intake would be best, based on health and medical history. A dry, scratchy throat is best alleviated using fruity hard candies as opposed to menthol lozenges, which have a drying effect.

Let's go through some foods that you or your loved one should avoid if there is a history of GERD or a voice disorder. Anyone with GERD should avoid spicy foods, which often result in acid flare-ups (heartburn). Foods that sound healthy, like citrus and acidic foods, such as lemons or tomatoes, can also be problematic for people with GERD, as they increase acid production. People have different reactions to milk and dairy products. Some people consume dairy products and have thickened mucus that causes them to cough or clear their throat. If that is the case, decrease dairy intake. Avoid, or at least minimize, intake of caffeinated foods and beverages. Caffeine works as a diuretic, which causes more frequent urination, which can cause dehydration. This can dry out the vocal cords, which can be a problem because your voice needs proper lubrication to work well. Most people cannot give up caffeine completely if it has been a staple of their diet, but consider consuming less coffee, caffeinated tea, and, sadly, chocolate, which also contains caffeine. Alcoholic beverages are drying and irritating to the vocal mechanism; drink two glasses of water for every drink containing alcohol that you consume. For hydration-conscious snacks, consider eating foods that naturally contain large amounts of water, such as watermelon, apples, pears, melons, grapes, and bell peppers.

Overall Health

The effects of illness or disease can be devastating to a person's voice. Overall, good health will support a stronger voice. If you find yourself with a cold or upper respiratory infection that affects your voice, try not to overuse it when you hear hoarseness. Today's technology allows us to have alternatives to speaking extensively. When your voice is affected by a cold or other illness, use email or text rather than talking on the phone. Overusing the voice when it is weak can lead to long-term voice problems. Many people think that whispering is resting their voice. But using a whisper puts more strain on your voice than speaking normally and should be avoided. The basic ideas of maintaining an overall healthy lifestyle will promote a stronger voice. It is important to eat a nutritious diet and maintain a healthy weight. Exercising to stay fit will help to ensure proper posture and efficient musculature, which will reduce stress and keep your voice sounding its best. Getting enough sleep is also a critical factor to staying healthy and maintaining our best selves.

The negative effects of smoking cannot be stated strongly enough. Don't smoke, or if you already do, please seek help to quit this deadly habit. Smoking increases the risk of throat and lung cancer greatly, and even secondhand smoke can be highly irritating to the vocal cords. Humidify your environment as needed, which can help combat the drying effects of the climate you live in or exposure to the dry air from air conditioning. Some over-the-counter cold or allergy medications can be drying. For example, long-term use of hormones may lower the pitch of a person's voice. Medications for allergies or colds, such as decongestants, can be drying on the tissue used to produce your voice. Speak with your physician if you experience voice changes or weakness that might be related to medications.

Healthy Voice Use

The way you use your voice has a lot to do with how you sound. Vocal hygiene is the inclusion of healthy voice habits and elimination of unhealthy behaviors that can be harmful to the structures that produce your voice.

Avoid yelling and screaming. If you are an excited sports fan or a teacher who needs to get the attention of your class, consider using a cowbell, whistle, or handclap rather than a loud voice. Coughing and throat clearing can be hard on the voice, as it causes our vocal cords to slam together. If these are habits for you, try to eliminate the source. For a dry throat, try drinking more water and using hard candies. For allergies, seek medical treatment so that you can eliminate the source of the postnasal drip. Many people with voice problems have behaviors that we can describe as "vocal abuse." If your job or hobbies require you to talk for long periods, be sure to take voice breaks, when you stop talking for at least ten minutes every two hours. It is nearly impossible to stop talking completely, which some people call "vocal rest." But you can incorporate "voice naps" into your daily routine by setting aside short periods when you do not use your voice. If you must communicate in a noisy environment, consider using amplification so you aren't straining to be louder. If you need to speak to someone who isn't nearby, move closer to that person rather than yelling across the room. If your spouse or communication partner has a hearing impairment, have them see an audiologist to address that problem rather than raising your voice. If you are sick or tired and your voice sounds hoarse, listen to what your body is telling you and do not overuse your voice. Doing so can cause much more serious voice problems as your body compensates in negative ways to perform. Always seek help from a physician or SLP if voice problems persist. The suggestions here are general, but SLPs work with voice clients to develop programs aimed at their specific needs and issues to improve their voice. It can be useful to have a specialist come up with a treatment plan that is tailored to a person's life and needs. You don't have to resign yourself to having a voice that sounds different as a result of aging or most other problems. Speech-language pathologists have many options that can help you keep your voice sounding young and strong.

What if My Voice Changes Following Surgery?

Many people experience voice changes after they have surgery, for two major reasons. The first is that some common types of surgery occur in the area of your throat and chest. Examples of these include cardiac and thyroid procedures. One of the important nerves that provides a message to help move our vocal cords travels long distances in the body and extends from the neck area all the way down and around the heart and then back up toward the neck. This specific nerve (the vagus nerve) is vulnerable to damage, like small nicks or abrasions that could occur during surgery. People who have this type of damage will sound breathy, as one of the vocal cords may not be moving as well as it should.

Another reason people have voice changes after surgery has to do with what medical personnel do to help you stay safe with your breathing during a surgical procedure. During all surgeries when a patient is under anesthesia, doctors intubate patients. This happens if the surgery is on your heart, your brain, or even your big toe! When a doctor intubates someone, a small plastic breathing tube is placed through the mouth and between the vocal cords, which are located in the windpipe, to help a person breathe during surgery. If you are having trouble picturing this, look at these structures in the illustration in appendix A. In some patients, the windpipe or vocal cords can become irritated and inflamed from this tube, which will cause the voice to sound different. Normally when this happens, people notice a breathy, weak, or hoarse voice. A person might complain of a sore throat when talking or swallowing, dryness, or feeling a constant need to clear their throat. Most of the time, the voice will improve back to normal function within several weeks, as long as the person is taking care of their voice (see the information in this chapter regarding safe voice use). If the voice problems last longer than two weeks, the individual should see an ENT to determine if they need medical intervention.

What Are the Effects of Neurological Issues on the Voice?

The issues previously mentioned in this chapter can affect caregivers and patients. This next section covers voice problems specific to people who have acquired brain injuries or degenerative diseases. These people need to express themselves to their best ability since it is critical that doctors and caregivers know if they are in pain or need help to get their basic needs met. If individuals with neurological issues experience voice problems, it is important that they see an ENT. This doctor will use a scope that goes through either the mouth or the nose to see the movements of the vocal cords. This procedure is not painful and will allow the ENT to determine the best way to treat the voice disorder.

Stroke

The issues that people have following a stroke depend very much on exactly which parts of the brain sustained damage during the event. As discussed in other chapters, a stroke can greatly affect speech, language, and swallowing (chapters 2, 4, and 5). During a stroke, there can also be specific damage to the nerves that help move our vocal cords, which can cause paralysis (total loss of movement) or paresis (weakness) of one or both cords. Depending on the damage, this can cause a voice to sound breathy and weak or hoarse and harsh. Following a stroke, many patients experience spontaneous recovery, when the brain, nerves, and muscles may improve and recover some lost function. While this may mean that voice problems noted early on will resolve partially or completely on their own, talk to your doctor or see an ENT if your loved one's voice is affected by a stroke. The information covered in chapter 4 on swallowing disorders shows that the vocal cords help to protect our airway from food and liquid (aspiration). A person who has vocal changes following a stroke could also have swallowing issues, often heard as a gurgly or wet-sounding voice when eating. An ENT who determines that a person has paralysis or paresis of the vocal cords can refer the patient to an SLP to improve movements of those cords. This may include exercises to improve the closure of the vocal cords (strengthening) or exercises to reduce tension (relaxation). Medical options for treatment might include injection of a filler to "fatten up" a paralyzed vocal cord or surgery to physically move the location of a vocal cord that isn't moving as it should. In extreme cases, both vocal cords can be paralyzed in a closed position, which does not allow the person to breathe well. This would likely result in a doctor performing a tracheostomy, which is a small incision, or cut, in the front of the neck through which the doctor makes an opening into the windpipe, or trachea. They insert a breathing tube that allows the person to breathe. This is an emergency procedure, and the person's voice would be a secondary concern, with the primary issue being their ability to breathe.

Parkinson's Disease

Parkinson's disease (PD) affects movement in two different ways. One effect is difficulty starting movements. When they take place, they are often slower and smaller than usual. An almost opposite effect due to damage to the brain occurs when people with PD have extra or unintended movements. Both impacts can cause a person with PD to experience challenges with their voice. The small, slow movements result in a quiet, breathy voice, and people with PD may find that their voice frequently fatigues easily. The result of extra movements can cause repetition of syllables (almost a stuttering-like behavior) and an occasional tremor in the voice. Fortunately, medications such as Levodopa or Sinemet can help people with PD experience more normal types of movements. There are two important things to know about these and other medications used to treat PD, though. First, many patients experience relief from movement issues when they first take PD medications, but the impact of the medication may lessen over time. Remember that PD is a degenerative brain disease, which means that a person with PD experiences a steady decline in movements. Also, some medications that help people with PD move their arms, legs, and trunk more normally have been shown to have no positive impact, or at times, even a negative impact, on speech, voice, and swallowing in those who have PD. So, it's important to remember that the effects of medication may or may not be helpful with voice, depending on the person and their situation. Speech therapy can be useful for people with PD in improving their ability to communicate. SLPs use many treatment techniques to address voice problems related to PD, including two that were designed specifically for use with those who have PD. Lee Silverman Voice Treatment (LSVT) focuses specifically on creating a louder voice, which is often the issue for these individuals. SLPs must attend a specialized training to become certified to use LSVT with patients. This treatment is intensive and involves four days of therapy per week for four weeks. There is also a fair amount of homework involved. For more information, please see the resource list for the LSVT website at the end of this chapter. Another type of treatment developed by the Parkinson Voice Project to improve vocal loudness is SPEAK OUT! / LOUD Crowd. In the first part of this training, SPEAK OUT!, individuals attend twelve speech therapy sessions, where they work with a trained SLP on voice, speech, and cognitive activities. There is a workbook for patients to use in these sessions and at home. At the end of that training, patients attend group sessions called LOUD Crowd, which are formatted to help people with a progressive disease like PD maintain their loud, understandable voice through speaking and singing activities. Please see the resource list at the end of this chapter for more information and to find where to attend SPEAK OUT! / LOUD Crowd sessions. One last point to remember is that all the safe vocal strategies mentioned in this chapter apply to people dealing with PD.

Vocal Tremor

A common neurological condition that can affect the voice is benign essential tremor (also called vocal tremor if it affects the voice). Signs can include tremor in the hands and head, as well as a shaky, or tremulous, voice. People can develop tremors in different parts of their body, but when muscles and structures that help us speak are trembling, then the voice can sound very shaky. This type of tremor can be inherited genetically, and we also find it more commonly in the aging population. When the person is speaking normally, some tremor can get "hidden" in all the speech sounds. Often, the tremor is much more easily heard if the person holds out long vowel sounds, like "aaaaah." If a tremor is noted in someone's voice, seeing a medical doctor is important. A neurologist will most likely diagnose the cause of a vocal tremor. It is possible that medical treatment can alleviate the tremor. Most commonly, an injection of botulinum toxin (Botox) into sections of the larynx can inhibit the muscles from causing extra movements, which can be helpful in some people. Every few months, these injections must be readministered. While an SLP cannot change what is going on neurologically, the patient can change their voice in some ways through speech therapy sessions. The resource list at the end of this chapter contains an excellent website for information on vocal tremor.

Other Neurogenic Voice Disorders

Other diseases and disorders related to the brain can cause difficulties with a person's voice. It is important to remember that people dealing with these types of voice disorders should see a neurologist or an ENT. Medical intervention can relieve or reduce some voice problems, and most times, an SLP can develop a treatment plan that will improve the voice.

Spasmodic dysphonia (SD) is an uncommon voice disorder where a person has spasming (sudden, involuntary muscle contractions) that occurs in the larynx and vocal cords. Depending on whether the spasms occur when the vocal cords are open or closed, the person's voice can sound breathy or harsh. Injections of Botox can be a useful treatment, and speech therapy may improve the voice of some people. A support group is an important recommendation for individuals dealing with SD. This condition can make it difficult to be understood. Speaking with SD can require a great deal of effort. Please see the resource list at the end of this chapter for more information.

Myasthenia gravis (MG) is a brain disease that can affect the muscles related to breathing. MG results in muscles that are weak and fatigue easily. Since breathing is such an important component in our voice, people with MG may develop voice problems early in the disease process. Sometimes, the first sign or symptom of a problem with MG is a voice issue. Commonly, patients with MG experience a softer voice than usual, breathiness, and a nasal-sounding voice. A neurologist will diagnose and treat people with MG, who generally respond well to medication.

Amyotrophic lateral sclerosis (ALS), commonly known as Lou Gehrig's disease, affects the nerves in the brain and spinal cord, resulting in weakness in all muscles in the body. While some patients develop symptoms initially in the limbs, others may have their first problems related to speech, voice, and swallowing. Eventually, all areas of the body will be affected as the disease progresses. People with ALS commonly have severe respiratory issues that impact the voice. They may sound breathy and nasally, and their voice may fatigue easily. Most people who have ALS will need to rely on a ventilator to breathe for them and may need a device to help them speak as the disease progresses. An SLP has many strategies to help the person with ALS feel more comfortable using their voice. You can find more information on this topic in chapter 2. Also, if the person will need a device to help them speak later in the disease process, it is important for that work to begin before they actually need it. This allows the SLP to communicate easily with the person while teaching them how to use the equipment. In addition, many of these devices can now use the person's own voice, as opposed to a robotic-sounding voice. This involves "banking" the person's voice by having the SLP record them saying words and sentences that can be put into the device. Then, if the person can no longer speak, they can press a key on the device to activate the desired word or sentence.

Traumatic brain injury (TBI) occurs when external forces result in brain damage. TBIs typically result from car accidents, falls, or explosions. People who have a TBI can have a wide range of difficulties, ranging from mild to severe in many or just a few areas. Respiratory issues are a common reason for voice problems in people with a TBI, and many have a tracheostomy at some point during treatment. A team of medical professionals will follow these individuals, with an SLP managing any communication or swallowing issues. People who have a TBI can learn strategies to help use their voice in the most effective manner.

What Is the Impact of a Voice Disorder?

Dealing with a voice that is suddenly or gradually different can be difficult. People who are not easily heard or understood can become frustrated when communicating with others. They may find it easier to isolate themselves from people they usually interact with, and this can lead to negative feelings, even depression. As a caregiver, your voice is critical to interacting with your loved one and with medical professionals on their behalf. If your loved one is dealing with a voice disorder, you will surely notice if they are not communicating effectively. Staying active and communicating with other people helps maintain our mental and emotional functioning. So it is critical to keep everyone's voices strong and healthy. Here are some important warning signs for caregivers. Be sure to seek medical assistance immediately if you see or hear any of the following:

- Hoarse voice that lasts longer than two weeks
- Voice changes with choking or difficulty swallowing
- Voice changes with any bleeding in the mouth or throat
- Voice changes with difficulty breathing

What Are the Important Take-Home Points in This Chapter?

- The voice is produced using air through the lungs, which makes the vocal cords vibrate into a sound that is then shaped by the nose and mouth.

- If neurological issues affect the parts of the body that help us produce voice, we may experience voice disorders.

- If we don't take care of our voice, we can develop voice disorders or make them worse.

- What we eat and drink and how we take care of overall health can affect our voice.

- Changes in the voice related to age are sometimes normal, but see an SLP to determine if there is another cause and if therapy will help.

- You should always see a doctor if you have pain or changes in your voice that last more than two weeks or if your voice interferes with your ability to communicate.

Remember, a person's voice helps communicate their thoughts and needs, but it also gives us a window into how they are feeling physically. Treatment from an ENT or SLP can often help with voice difficulties. So, as a caregiver, seek help for yourself or your loved one as needed for any voice symptoms. Our voices are worth protecting.

REFERENCES

Basaraba, S. (2020, February 4). *5 ways our voices change as we age.* Very Well Health. https://www.verywellhealth.com/ways-voices-change-as-we-age-2223342.

Boone, D. R., McFarlane, S. C., Von Berg, S. L., & Zraick, R. I. (2014). *The voice and voice therapy* (9th ed.). Pearson Education.

Linville, S. E. (2001). *Vocal aging*. Singular Thomson Learning.

RESOURCES

ALS Association: https://www.als.org/

International Essential Tremor Foundation: https://www.essentialtremor.org

Vocal Tremor: https://www.essentialtremor.org/wp-content/uploads/2014/05/TremorTalkApril2014FINAL.pdf

Lee Silverman Voice Treatment (LSVT): https://www.lsvtglobal.com/

Myasthenia Gravis Foundation of America: http://myasthenia.org/

Parkinson Foundation Helpline: 1-800-473-4636 to help locate an SLP in your area.

Parkinson Voice Project: https://www.parkinsonvoiceproject.org

SPEAK OUT!/LOUD Crowd Programs: https://www.parkinsonvoiceproject.org/SPEAKOUT

National Spasmodic Dysphonia Association (support groups): https://www.dysphonia.org/

UT Voice Center San Antonio: https://lsom.uthscsa.edu/otolaryngology/centers/ut-voice-center/

Voice Care: https://lsom.uthscsa.edu/otolaryngology/centers/ut-voice-center/voice-care/

ABOUT THE AUTHOR

Dr. Connie Porcaro is an Associate Professor in the Department of Communication Sciences and Disorders at Florida Atlantic University (FAU). She received her BA in Communication Sciences and Disorders from the University of South Dakota, her MA in Speech Pathology from the University of Northern Colorado, and her PhD in Speech and Hearing Sciences from the University of Arizona. Dr. Porcaro instructs courses at FAU covering voice, speech, and swallowing disorders in adults. She lectures annually for the FAU Charles E. Schmidt College of Medicine on the topics of adult neurogenic communication disorders.

Dr. Porcaro is certified by the American Speech-Language-Hearing Association and has worked as a speech-language pathologist for more than twenty-five years with clients of all ages. Her primary area of research has focused on intelligibility in patients with speech and voice disorders and how speakers can improve communication with their listeners. She has published research articles in top journals, including the *American Journal of Speech-Language Pathology* and the *International Journal of Speech-Language Pathology*. Dr. Porcaro is a frequent presenter at the Annual Convention of the American Speech-Language- Hearing Association and often presents for state association conventions as an invited speaker. She is an active member of the Leadership Team Professional Development Subcommittee for the American Speech-Language-Hearing Association Special Interest Group on Neurophysiology and Neurogenic Speech and Language Disorders. She has received grant funding from the FAU Healthy Aging Research Initiative to investigate voice and swallowing changes in healthy elderly participants. Dr. Porcaro has received grant funding from the Parkinson Voice Project to facilitate training for graduate students who provide free speech therapy for individuals with Parkinson's disease.

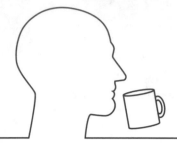

FOUR

A Tough Pill to Swallow

Maintaining Good Nutrition When Swallowing Is Difficult

Barbara O'Connor Wells, PhD, CCC-SLP,
and Marissa A. Barrera, PhD, MSCS, CCC-SLP

Fred was recently diagnosed with ALS. His wife, Mary, has done lots of reading about this disease and what to expect as it progresses. She has been noticing that Fred is eating and drinking less and less. His energy level is low, and he gets fatigued easily. She thinks he looks thinner too. When he eats and drinks, she notices some concerning things. He takes a very long time to chew and swallow his food. He has been coughing and clearing his throat a lot, particularly when he drinks his favorite beverages, like his morning coffee and juice. One time, he choked on a piece of chicken, and she nearly had to call 911. "Time to discuss these swallow problems with Dr. Jones," she thinks. She picks up the phone to make an appointment for early next week.

Eva is a 75-year-old widow, with no known medical conditions. She has been having difficulty swallowing for about six months. At first, she experienced trouble swallowing solid foods, but over the last few weeks, swallowing liquids has also become challenging. Mealtimes are now stressful. Eva avoids certain types of foods, such as meat and stews, because she is fearful of the food going down the wrong pipe. From time to time, she has

the sensation of food caught in her throat and tightness in her chest. With-
out intentional dieting, Eva has lost eight pounds over the last six months.
Instead of enjoying her retirement, Eva is worried every time she sits down
at her kitchen table and is embarrassed to eat out with her friends.

Why Swallowing?

If you are reading this chapter, you may be caring for a person who
is having trouble swallowing. It is important that our book include a
chapter devoted to swallowing problems because acquired brain injuries, degenerative diseases, and other disorders can result in difficulty
swallowing. In addition, our risk for swallowing problems increases
as we age. Safe and efficient swallowing is at the heart of good nutrition and hydration, which are essential for overall health, happiness,
and wellness.

We want to stress that this chapter is a basic overview of this
topic. If your loved one is showing signs and symptoms of a swallowing problem, it is imperative that you seek the medical expertise of
a licensed speech-language pathologist (SLP) who specializes in this
area, or a physician.

What Is Dysphagia?

You may have heard the term *dysphagia* (pronounced "dis-fay-ja")
from physicians, nurses, SLPs, or other medical staff. This term means
difficulty swallowing. According Groher and Crary (2021) and the
National Foundation of Swallowing Disorders (https://swallowing
disorderfoundation.com), between 300,000 and 600,000 individuals are newly diagnosed with dysphagia each year in the United
States. Because of advances in medical technology and increases in
life expectancy, the risk for developing dysphagia as we age is steadily
increasing.

Dysphagia is not a disease but rather a symptom of underlying disease (Groher & Crary, 2021). Swallowing difficulty is caused by something else, such as a stroke, traumatic brain injury (TBI), or degenerative diseases like Parkinson's disease or amyotrophic lateral sclerosis (ALS, or Lou Gehrig's disease).

Dysphagia is a serious medical issue that can cause dehydration (not getting enough fluids, like water), malnutrition (poor, imbalanced diet), confusion, change in medical status, and a serious medical consequence called aspiration pneumonia. This is a type of pneumonia that occurs when food and liquids go down the wrong pipe and end up in the lungs instead of the stomach. Aspiration pneumonia is a leading cause of death in some medical conditions, like Parkinson's disease (Barrera & O'Connor Wells, 2019).

What Are Some Common Causes of Dysphagia?

Swallowing problems can have many causes. It is beyond this chapter to provide a full list. Here, we highlight some common ones, grouped into five major categories: (1) neurological causes, (2) obstructions in the swallowing pathway, (3) respiratory conditions, (4) aging, and (5) medications. It's important to remember that there are about fifty pairs of muscles and several nerves that deal with swallowing (NIDCD, 2017). These muscles can become weak, rigid, or uncoordinated, just as arms and legs can. We also must remember that we stop breathing when we swallow, so that the food or liquid can go down the right way. Therefore, if someone is having trouble breathing, then swallowing may also be a problem.

Neurological Causes

Damage to the nervous system (brain, nerves, and spinal cord) can affect the nerves and muscles responsible for swallowing. This can lead to dysphagia. Some common neurological causes of dysphagia include strokes, brain tumors, traumatic brain injuries (TBIs), Parkinson's disease, multiple sclerosis (MS), and dementia. In the case study about *Fred* at the beginning of this chapter, for example, his ALS (or Lou Gehrig's disease) caused his swallowing problems.

Obstructions in the Swallowing Pathway

An obstruction or narrowing in the throat or esophagus can prevent the passage of food and liquid and make swallowing difficult. *Eva*, in the second story at the beginning of this chapter, was complaining of food getting stuck, which may suggest an obstruction or inflammation. Some causes include cancer (oral cancer, laryngeal cancer, esophageal cancer), pharyngeal (throat) pouches (also known as Zenker's diverticulum), allergic esophagitis (an inflammation in the esophagus usually caused by reflux), radiation treatment, and infections. Dysphagia can also develop as a complication of head or neck surgery.

Respiratory Conditions

Respiratory diseases, such as chronic obstructive pulmonary disease (COPD), asthma, emphysema, and chronic bronchitis can affect the coordination between breathing and swallowing. If someone has a respiratory problem, they may try to breathe while swallowing, resulting in food or liquid going down the wrong pipe.

Aging

Presbyphagia, or expected changes in swallowing associated with normal aging, can affect swallowing safety. These changes can include things like less tongue strength for moving the food around in the mouth, which can cause food residue in the mouth after the swallow. The result may be taking too long to swallow, which can make an older adult more prone to coughing and choking. Although age-related changes in swallowing can increase the risk for developing dysphagia, the swallowing skills of an older adult are not necessarily impaired. Because this is an important topic, additional information on presbyphagia appears later in this chapter.

Medications

An important but often unrecognized cause of dysphagia is medication. Dysphagia can result as a drug side effect. For example, some medicines may make the mouth too dry or may increase the amount of saliva in the mouth. These can affect how food and liquid moves through the different phases of the swallow. Common classes of medications that may cause dysphagia include (1) antipsychotics, (2) antidepressants, (3) anticonvulsants, (4) analgesics, and (5) anxiolytics. If you have a concern that your loved one's medications may affect their swallowing safety, please consult with a physician or pharmacist.

What Are Some Signs and Symptoms of Dysphagia?

The medical team, particularly the SLP, may talk about different *signs* or *symptoms* of dysphagia. If your loved one has any of these issues, this may mean a possible dysphagia:

- Coughing, choking, or gagging on food or liquid
- Frequent throat clearing while eating or drinking
- Drooling or difficulty controlling saliva
- Recent bouts of aspiration pneumonia (when saliva, food, or drink enters the lungs, causing a serious lung infection)
- A history of frequent temperature spikes
- Gurgled-sounding or wet breathing after eating or drinking
- Regurgitation, or reflux, of food or liquid (coming back up into the throat)

- Frequent heartburn and need to use antacids

- Hoarse or wet and gurgly voice

- Pain when swallowing (odynophagia)

- Unexplained and undesired weight loss

- Difficulty starting the swallow and "getting going"

- Feeling food or liquid get stuck

What Are the Stages of Swallowing and What's Normal versus Abnormal?

In a healthy individual, swallowing is a coordinated and fast process. We swallow close to one thousand times a day, even when sleeping, but rarely have to think about it. It is normal for liquids to go down faster than foods, since liquids do not require chewing. It is also normal for different foods to vary in how long we need to chew and swallow them, depending on their texture, taste, and temperature. For example, we swallow a spoonful of applesauce much quicker than a piece of meat. Also, we swallow differently depending on how we consume the food or liquid. For example, we may swallow a small sip of liquid from a cup quicker than multiple sips of that same liquid through a straw. It is also normal, as we age, for meals to take longer and for us to eat smaller, more frequent meals.

Oral Stage

Now, imagine you have taken a bite of your favorite meal. When you take that first bite, your lips come together to create a seal as you take the food off the fork or spoon or take a sip of a liquid from the rim of the cup. This is the beginning of the oral (mouth) stage of swallowing. In this first stage, food or liquid mixes with the saliva in your mouth. As food is chewed, the jaw makes a side-to-side motion, and the tongue moves similarly. These movements of the jaw and tongue create a cohesive "ball" that is ready for swallowing, known as a *bolus*. A bolus can be food, liquid, saliva, or a pill. If your loved one has difficulty in the oral stage of swallowing, they may pocket food in the cheeks or have difficulty chewing food. These difficulties may result from weakness of the tongue or the face muscles. Also, the food or liquid may drool out of the mouth if the lips are not strong. This part of the oral stage can take as long as needed and will vary, depending on what type of food or liquid was placed in the mouth. For example, it will take much longer to form a bolus when chewing a piece of steak than with a sip of water.

After a bolus is made, chewing stops and the tongue lifts up and moves the bolus to the back of the mouth. This process is also part of the oral stage of swallowing. Try swallowing right now and you will feel your tongue push against the roof of your mouth, which pushes the saliva toward the back. A person with dysphagia may have slow or weak muscle movements for pushing the bolus to the back of their mouth. This can lead to a delay in starting the next stage of swallow and food or liquid being left behind in the mouth (residue). This residue is typically inside the cheeks, under the tongue, or on the tongue. It is important for your loved one to be aware of this residue and try to swallow it again or take a drink to help wash it down. A finger can also be used to clear this residue.

Pharyngeal Stage

In the pharyngeal (throat) stage of swallowing, the bolus moves to the back of the mouth and enters the upper section of the throat (pharynx). The entrance to the airway (windpipe) is protected from the bolus entering by several muscle movements. For example, the vocal cords close together, which helps to keep the bolus out of the airway. Breathing stops for a short time when our vocal cords are closed. Try swallowing one more time now and put your hand gently on the front of your neck. You should feel a slight lifting of your Adam's apple. This helps keep the bolus moving the way it should, toward the esophagus. The pharyngeal (throat) muscles contract and squeeze the bolus down toward the esophagus (food tube).

Various things can go wrong in the pharyngeal stage of swallowing. A delay in the swallow can throw off the timing of this stage. You may observe choking, clearing of the throat, or coughing during meals. A person with dysphagia may have difficulty coordinating the muscles and movements for swallowing. This can cause the bolus to enter the nose, sit on top of the airway, or accidentally enter the lungs, which can lead to a serious medical condition, called aspiration pneumonia. Aspiration occurs when saliva, food, or drink enters the voice box, windpipe, or lungs. This is colloquially referred to as something going down the wrong pipe.

Esophageal Stage

In the last stage of swallowing, known as the esophageal stage, the bolus reaches the esophagus, which is a muscular tube that begins in the pharynx (throat) and leads to the stomach. The muscles in the esophagus contract like a wave to move the food or liquid from the top of the esophagus to the bottom, and then into the stomach. This should normally take between 8 and 20 seconds. But things can also go wrong in the esophagus. With aging, there may be changes in the esophageal muscles. This can lead to increased chances for the bolus to get stuck (as in the case of *Eva*), or come back up after going into the stomach (reflux). In this last stage of swallowing, your loved one may complain of feeling food or liquid get stuck in their chest or of feeling reflux (the food or liquid coming back up). This stage of the swallow will often involve the expertise of a gastroenterologist, or GI doctor. A gastroenterologist is a medical doctor who specializes in diagnosing and treating diseases or disorders of the digestive system, which includes the esophagus and stomach. To confirm problems in this stage of the swallow, the SLP will rely on the expertise of the GI doctor, who will use imaging technology, such as an upper GI series or barium esophagram, to examine the gastrointestinal system of a person.

In short, the act of enjoying your favorite meal is a complex process that involves about fifty pairs of muscles and several nerves. Any problems along the way can lead to signs and symptoms of dysphagia. For a helpful visual of the swallowing anatomy, please see appendix C at the end of this book.

How Does Aging Affect Swallowing?

As we age, changes happen that can affect the way we live. For example, one may develop presbycusis, where hearing diminishes with age, or presbyopia, where vision worsens (see chapters 1 and 3). Age-related changes can also affect our swallow, referred to as *presbyphagia*. These are relatively normal changes in swallowing that occur with age and should not cause aspiration (Barrera & O'Connor Wells, 2019; McCoy & Desai, 2018) or other swallowing-related complaints. Individuals who have normal, age-related changes to swallowing can still eat and drink safely. Taste sensation can also change, as does olfaction (smell), so foods and liquids may not have the same appeal as they previously did. With age also comes a reduction in the elasticity and strength of our muscles and overall muscle mass. We call this *sarcopenia*. Because we use many muscles to swallow, normal aging may also affect these muscles. For example, the oral phase of swallowing may take longer because the tongue is not as strong as it used to be. It may take more effort to push the food or liquids back to swallow. This can lead to things like a longer time for chewing or food being left behind in the mouth after the swallow. There may be a slightly longer time for a swallow to occur. Older persons may change their diet and avoid foods they find difficult to chew and swallow, such as tough meats. In addition, they may be more prone to feeling the food and liquid coming back up (reflux).

How Is Swallowing Evaluated?

If dysphagia is suspected, the physician or medical team may send a consultation to an SLP for a swallowing evaluation. The first step would typically be a clinical swallow evaluation (CSE). The SLP can complete the evaluation at the bedside, at home, or in a private office. During a CSE, a review of the medical chart is completed. The SLP is seeking information to help determine the causes of the swallowing issue. For example, the SLP may look for things like a family history of dysphagia, previous swallow evaluations, lung or pulmonary history, and neurological history. The evaluation will include an interview of your loved one (if applicable), their family members and caregivers, and the medical team. The SLP will ask about things like allergies, current foods and liquids that your loved one eats and drinks, if there is a history of pneumonia, frequency of the problem, and so forth.

Your loved one will then undergo an evaluation of their oral muscles. This will involve checking the movement, range of motion, coordination, and strength for the lips, tongue, cheeks, and jaw, and looking at overall facial appearance. The SLP will also complete an examination of the inside of the mouth to check salivation status, oral hygiene, and movement of the soft palate. For the oral muscles, the SLP may ask your loved one to "smile," "pucker your lips," "stick out your tongue," "move your tongue side to side," along with various other movements. The goal here is to see how these muscles move and to learn about the overall sensation. A screening of language and cognition (for example, memory, attention, comprehension) will also take place to ensure your loved one is alert and awake enough to take part in the evaluation. You would never want to feed someone if they are too tired or sleeping! Other cognitive areas assessed include attention, ability to follow simple directions, simple naming of common objects, and some questions to assess memory (for example, "What's your doctor's name?" "Where were you born?").

Next, the SLP may perform a quick voice assessment. They will ask your loved one to say "ah" and will listen to the clarity and quality of the voice. For example, it would be a concern if your loved one could not produce their voice when asked; this could mean that the vocal cords are not working properly. Or, if their voice sounded low or wet, this could mean that some food or liquid may be in the voice box (larynx). The SLP will also want to see if your loved one can clear their throat or cough when told to do so and will also check the health of the gums and teeth.

If it's appropriate, the SLP will then give different food and liquid textures to assess the swallow. This may include regular food (for example, cookie or cracker), soft solid (for example, pasta, banana), mechanical soft (such as scrambled eggs), pureed food (applesauce, pudding), and then liquids (water thin, nectar thick, or honey thick).

When signs or symptoms of pharyngeal (throat-level) swallowing issues are observed, the SLP will need to conduct further testing to best understand the muscle performance (physiology) during the swallow. When that is the case, the SLP will ask for either an X-ray swallow study or an endoscopic swallow study.

The X-ray swallow study is called a modified barium swallow (MBS) study, or videofluoroscopy. This involves your loved one having an X-ray while eating and drinking. A radiologist is a medical doctor who specializes in diagnosing and treating injuries, diseases, and disorders using imaging technology (i.e., radiology). During an MBS, the radiologist operates the fluoroscopy machine to take moving images (X-rays) of a person while they are swallowing foods and liquids.

The SLP will prepare different food and liquid textures for the study. They mix these foods and liquids with a special product called barium. This makes the food and liquid visible during the X-ray study; the bolus will show up black so that the SLP and radiologist can see it move as the person swallows it. During the study, your loved one will sit in a special chair, comfortably, in the fluoroscopy suite. The SLP will feed them food and liquids, or your loved one may feed themselves. During each bite or sip, the radiologist will turn on the machine, and the swallow will be visible as a moving X-ray. The SLP will view your loved one's mouth to see how the tongue moves for chewing, and into the throat to see how the swallow happens and if there's anything left behind or that ends up going into the windpipe. The SLP will also be able to see the food or liquid enter the esophagus and move down into the stomach. If reflux occurs, the SLP and radiologist may observe it (although this test is not the best for diagnosing reflux). After the MBS study, the SLP and radiologist will discuss the findings and come up with a diagnosis and recommendations.

Fiberoptic endoscopic evaluation of swallowing, or FEES, is another form of evaluation for dysphagia. Unlike the MBS, which involves a trip to radiology and minor exposure to radiation, FEES uses an endoscope, which is a long, thin, and flexible instrument with a camera in it, and can be done anywhere—at the patient's bedside, home, or in the SLP's office. The scope is passed through the nose and down the throat to see the swallow. The SLP or otolaryngologist will pass a scope in one nostril. An otolaryngologist, also commonly called an ear, nose, and throat (ENT) doctor, is a physician who specializes in diagnosing and treating injuries, diseases, or disorders of the ear, nose, or throat. In terms of a FEES procedure, the ENT may be the professional who puts the scope through your loved one's nose and throat to test the swallow. The scope moves through the nose until it reaches the back wall of the throat (pharynx); then, the scope travels downward until the SLP or ENT can see the vocal cords and voice box. Once the scope is in place, the SLP or ENT will have your loved one eat and drink various foods and liquids. Food coloring (usually green or blue) is used to dye foods or liquids so that they are visible during the FEES. Just like during the MBS, the SLP and ENT will present one texture at a time and make observations and recommendations.

During the FEES, the SLP will look closely at how the vocal cords move. Remember, to protect the lungs from aspiration, the vocal cords need to come together and close. Also, if there is an issue with vocal cord closure, you will hear it in the person's voice (they may sound hoarse or breathy or may not have any voice). During the FEES, the SLP will look at how well the food or liquid clears after each swallow. If lots of green or blue dye remains in the throat area, this can mean that sensation is not good; also, any food or liquid left behind can later be aspirated into the lungs. For example, if your loved one were to take a nap after a meal, food or liquid residue could be aspirated later.

How Can Swallowing Problems Be Treated?

It is beyond the scope of this chapter to outline all the different treatment options for dysphagia. As a caregiver of a patient with dysphagia, it would be too overwhelming. What we would like for you to know is that there are two general approaches, or categories of treatment, for dysphagia: compensation and rehabilitation.

Compensation versus Rehabilitation

Compensations are strategies done during a meal to make your loved one eat and drink more safely. We consider compensations temporary. These strategies will not improve the muscles for swallowing or strengthen anything, but they allow the person with dysphagia to eat and drink more safely. Some well-known and frequently used compensations include postural changes and diet modifications. Postural changes might mean your loved one sits in a different position or holds their head differently when eating and drinking. If your loved one goes through an evaluation with an SLP, this specialist may recommend safe postural changes. One thing to always remember is that your loved one should be alert and sitting as close to 90 degrees upright as possible (or some other modification suggested by their physician or SLP). Diet changes are another form of compensation. These changes may include things such as eating blended or pureed food instead of solid foods or drinking liquids that are thicker. Besides diet changes, another recommendation may be special utensils or devices for eating or drinking (for example, special spoons, forks, cups, slip-free plates, or placemats) to help your loved one during mealtimes. The SLP will often work closely with an occupational therapist (OT) to decide if your loved one needs special devices for eating or drinking.

Rehabilitation, on the other hand, includes exercises if the SLP thinks the muscles for swallowing can improve. This may involve exercises to improve the muscles of the tongue and lips against resistance or performing hard or effortful swallows ("swallow like you are swallowing a golf ball and squeeze your muscles"). These are just a few examples.

Ultimately, the SLP will make the determination regarding which therapy approaches are best suited to your loved one's dysphagia symptoms. Treatment courses are individualized and include not only the SLP recommendations, but also your goals and the goals of your loved one. Achieving and maintaining good nutrition and hydration should be the driving force behind the approach to your loved one's dysphagia therapy. Sometimes, the swallow problem is severe and not responsive to treatment. At that point, the medical team may explore tube-feeding options and discuss those with you and your loved one. We discuss this topic later in this chapter.

What Are the Different Food and Liquid Textures and Commercially Available Thickeners?

After a SLP has evaluated your loved one's swallow, they may recommend changes in diet to help ensure safe and efficient swallowing. Diet changes, as previously mentioned, are a form of compensation. There are various types and textures that a person with dysphagia might be assessed for to determine which combination of food and liquid is the safest for them to eat and drink. In terms of foods, we have *regular* texture, which includes items like solid meats and hard foods, like pretzels. *Soft* texture includes food that requires some level of chewing but is not as tough as regular. Some examples include a banana or soft cookie. *Mechanical soft* means foods like mac and cheese, tuna salad, and scrambled eggs. And the least difficult to chew is *pureed* texture, which includes foods like smooth applesauce and pudding.

The SLP might recommend softer texture foods because they are easier for some people to chew and control in the mouth. For example, pureed food does not take much effort to chew and can be easily molded into a bolus. Most of your loved one's favorite foods can be pureed in a blender. Many commercially available blenders even have a "puree" setting.

In terms of beverages or drinks, we have *thin* liquids, which include water, coffee, most juices, and tea. The next step thicker is *nectar* liquid, which is like nectar or guava juice consistency. The thickest liquid is *honey*—this is as thick as its name. In certain cases, individuals should drink thicker liquids for safety reasons. They move slower, so we consider them safer because a person with dysphagia may control them better. Thicker liquids are less likely than thinner liquids to end up in the lungs.

It is important for you to be aware of the International Dysphagia Diet Standardisation Initiative (IDDSI), which began in early

2016. The IDDSI is a task force made up of experts in the topic of swallowing disorders and nutrition from around the world. The goal of this task force is to make sure that what we call pureed food or moderately thick liquid is the same for SLPs, medical professionals, persons with dysphagia, and caregivers in other parts of the world. The IDDSI created an "eight-level continuum of liquid (drinks) and solid (food) consistencies" (Piera & Rioles, 2019, 38). For more information on IDDSI, please consult your loved one's SLP and the IDDSI website (https://iddsi.org/).

To make a beverage nectar or honey thick, there are commercially available thickening agents. These are starch based or xanthan gum based, and they can be added to any beverage to make them nectar or honey consistency. Thickening agents are used to help patients gain more control over their liquids when they swallow them. Thickening agents also help reduce the chances of the liquid getting into the lungs. A few common examples of these include: Thick & Easy, Thick-It, Thik & Clear, SimplyThick, and Resource ThickenUp. You can add them to either hot or cold beverages. They are tasteless and odorless and should not change the flavor or smell of the liquid. You can purchase thickening agents at your local pharmacy or online. There are specific instructions on the container about how to thicken your loved one's liquids. The instructions will tell you how many teaspoons or packets of thickener to mix with specific ounces of fluid. It is important to read the instructions carefully and ask the SLP or nurse for training before your loved one is discharged home. A final point on thickening agents: it is important to allow the beverage to thicken before drinking, but don't let it sit for too long because that could change the thickness. Make sure the liquid mixes well with the thickener to avoid lumps.

In short, it is important to remember that dietary changes should be made only after an SLP has completed a swallowing evaluation and determined which diet is safest for your loved one. If a modified diet is recommended for your loved one, be sure the SLP trains you on how to mix liquids to make them thicker and that you learn about what food options are available. SLPs know that it is a challenge to balance these recommended diet changes with making the new textures of food or liquids appealing and satisfying to your loved one. Sometimes, you can mold foods to look like their original texture (for example, taking pureed beef and molding it to look like a hamburger patty) or add seasoning to enhance the flavor.

What if My Loved One Cannot Eat and Drink Anymore? What Are Feeding Tubes?

If the swallowing problem is severe and does not improve with compensations or treatment, the recommendation may be NPO, or no food or liquid by mouth. The alternate way to receive nutrition and hydration would be from a feeding tube. We can't stress enough that a feeding tube is not a life sentence. For some patients, it is a temporary option that will help them stabilize and become strong enough to eat orally again (with dysphagia treatment from an SLP).

The first level of tube feeding may be a nasogastric tube (NGT). The tube is placed in the nose and goes directly down the esophagus and into the stomach. A liquid formula is placed through the tube, which contains all the nutrients your loved one needs. There are several different types of liquid tube-feeding formulas (for example, Osmolite, Jevity, Isosource, and Nutren). Your loved one's medical team will select the liquid formula most appropriate for your loved one, in conjunction with the recommendations of the dietitian. The NGT is typically only recommended for about 30 days. This type of feeding tube is easily reversed by the medical team by removing the tube from the nose. This does not require surgery. It can cause irritation to the nose and throat and may make your loved one more prone to reflux. To prevent reflux, the person receiving the tube feeding sits upright during and for approximately one hour after the feeding. Sometimes, a person with an NGT can still eat or drink select items if they have a small feeding tube. Your loved one's medical team makes that recommendation.

A surgically placed feeding tube is a more permanent option. There are some different types. Gastrostomy (*gastro* refers to stomach) tube (or G-tube) is a feeding tube that is placed in the stomach through the abdominal wall. The most common type of G-tube is a PEG. PEG means percutaneous (under the skin) endoscopic gastrostomy. This type of tube is usually placed during a relatively short and minor surgical procedure under local anesthesia. The liquid formula passes through the tube, bypassing the mouth, throat, and esophagus, and goes directly into the stomach. The hole where the tube goes through is called a *stoma*; it needs to be kept clean and sterile to prevent infection. The PEG can be reversed if your loved one shows improved swallowing.

Jejunostomy, or J-tube, is another surgically placed feeding tube. It is less common than the PEG. This tube goes directly into the jejunum, which is part of the small intestine. The J-tube bypasses the stomach completely, so it requires a special liquid formula. This tube reduces the risk for reflux and is a good option for anyone with issues in the stomach.

There are also forms of intravenous (IV) nutrition, where nutrition goes directly into the bloodstream. IV nutrition is recommended for a short time for individuals with serious medical issues. For more detailed information about tube feeding, please contact your loved one's physician or dietitian.

What Are Some Tips for Safe and Easy Swallowing?

- Only feed your loved one when they are alert and awake. Imagine trying to eat or drink when you are sleepy. Swallowing requires a person to be fully awake, alert, and engaged during a meal. If your loved one is drowsy, there is increased risk that they will choke during mealtime. Best to wait and try later, when he or she is fully engaged with you.

- Be sure your loved one is in a good posture for eating and drinking. Their elbows should rest on the table. This will keep the upper body and chest steady during the meal. Try to have your loved one sit as upright as possible. A 90-degree upright position is the best posture. Additionally, keep their feet firmly positioned on the floor or on the footrest of the wheelchair. Never have them eat or drink when lying back or down. If possible, sit your loved one in a chair instead of a bed during mealtime.

- It is important to practice good oral hygiene. Regular teeth brushing can reduce the chance of bacteria in the mouth, which can eventually make its way into the lungs and lead to pneumonia. If your loved one cannot to do this on their own, you might need to provide help. You should perform oral hygiene after each meal or snack.

- Be sure to clear food or liquid from the mouth before taking the next bite. It may be necessary to remind your loved one to clear any excess food before continuing with the meal. If you don't do this, it can lead to pocketing of food in the cheeks or on or under the tongue.

- When swallowing pills, if taking them with liquids is difficult, try mixing them into a small bowl of pudding, applesauce, or yogurt. Remember to check with your loved one's physician or pharmacist to see which medications can be crushed and taken with food. You can also try putting pills into a soft piece of cheese or bread.

- Alternate between food and drink. General rule of thumb: one sip of liquid for every three bites of food. This will help wash the food down with each sip of liquid and reduce the likelihood of food getting left behind in the mouth. Ask your loved one periodically if you can look into their mouth to check for food or liquid left behind. If you see anything, you can remind them to clear it with the tongue or a finger.

- Modify utensils and cups. Try using a straw for better control of liquids entering the mouth or eliminate the use of a straw if it is too difficult to control the flow and speed of liquids. Taking liquids by a spoon is also an option instead of drinking from a cup. Changing utensils may require some trial and error to figure out the best ones for your loved one to be safe during meals.

- Consider minimizing foods that combine two textures, such as selected soups and cereals that have both solid and liquid in one spoonful. These combined textures are complex and require more coordination than a single texture. A good example of a mixed texture is chicken noodle soup. The broth is a thin liquid; the noodles are mechanical soft; and the vegetables and chicken are regular texture.

- If your loved one gets food stuck in their throat, have them cough hard twice, followed by one hard, or effortful, swallow ("pretend like you are swallowing a big ball of food"). This may help remove the food stuck in the throat and move it along toward the food tube (esophagus).

- If your loved one is coughing or choking, do not offer liquids until they stop coughing or choking. Drinking something when you are already coughing and choking can make it much worse! Be sure to wait until they can talk comfortably again before giving anything more to eat or drink.

- Keeping a food and liquid journal is a great idea to help identify what foods and liquids are easy versus hard for your loved one. Identifying problem foods or liquids will be helpful information to provide to your loved one's physician and SLP. It will also have you and your loved one thinking more about swallowing and nutrition.

What Are the Important Take-Home Points in This Chapter?

- Dysphagia is the medical term for a swallowing problem.

- Dysphagia can lead to a serious medical condition called aspiration pneumonia.

- Safe swallowing involves the coordination of some fifty pairs of muscles and several nerves and takes place in three stages: oral, pharyngeal, and esophageal. Dysphagia can occur in one or all of these stages.

- The SLP is a swallowing expert who works closely with other professionals to diagnose dysphagia using either MBS or FEES.

- Swallowing problems can be improved or compensated for by swallowing therapy, conducted by an SLP.

- If your loved one cannot swallow food and liquids safely by mouth, the medical team may consider the need for a feeding tube.

In conclusion, we hope you have learned a lot of helpful information from this chapter on swallowing. Our goal is that this chapter has given you some "food for thought" and taught you about the importance of safe swallowing to maintain good nutrition and hydration.

REFERENCES

Barrera, M., & O'Connor Wells, B. (2019). Presbyphagia versus dysphagia: Normal versus abnormal swallowing symptoms in older adults with Parkinson disease and multiple sclerosis. *Topics in Geriatric Rehabilitation,* 35(3), 217–33.

Groher, M. E., & Crary, M. A. (2021). *Dysphagia: Clinical management in adults and children* (3rd ed.). Elsevier.

McCoy, Y. M., & Desai, R. V. (2018). Presbyphagia versus dysphagia: Identifying age-related changes in swallow function. *Perspectives,* 3(15), 15–21.

National Institute on Deafness and Other Communication Disorders (NIDCD). (2017, March 6). *Dysphagia.* https://www.nidcd.nih.gov/health/dysphagia

Piera, L., & Rioles, S. (2019). Developing an IDDSI-compliant dysphagia diet. *ASHA Leader,* 24(4), 38–40.

RESOURCES

American Gastroenterological Association: https://www.gastro.org/

American Speech-Language-Hearing Association: http://www.asha.org/

Centers for Disease Control and Prevention: http://www.cdc.gov/

EAT Bar: https://www.theeatbar.com/

International Dysphagia Diet Standardisation Initiative: https://iddsi.org/

Mayo Clinic: https://www.mayoclinic.org/

National Foundation of Swallowing Disorders: https://swallowingdisorderfoundation.com/

National Institute on Deafness and Other Communication Disorders (NIDCD): https://www.nidcd.nih.gov

Dysphagia: https://www.nidcd.nih.gov/health/dysphagia

Resource ThickenUp: http://www.nestlenutritionstore.com

SimplyThick: https://www.simplythick.com/

SwallowStudy.com: https://www.swallowstudy.com

Thick & Easy: http://www.hormelhealthlabs.com/

Thick-It: http://thickit.com/

Thik & Clear: https://www.alimed.com/thik-clear.html

ABOUT THE AUTHORS

Dr. Barbara O'Connor Wells is an Associate Professor and Clinical Supervisor in the Department of Speech-Language Pathology at Nova Southeastern University (NSU). She received her BA in Speech Pathology and Audiology and her MA in Speech-Language Pathology from St. John's University, New York, and her PhD in Speech-Language-Hearing Sciences from the Graduate Center of the City University of New York (CUNY). She teaches coursework and supervises individual and group treatment sessions in the areas of dysphagia, motor speech, and adult language disorders at NSU.

Dr. O'Connor Wells is certified by the American Speech-Language-Hearing Association (ASHA) and has twenty-five years of experience in acute, subacute, long-term, and homecare rehabilitation of adult neurogenic communication, cognition, and swallowing disorders. She is licensed in both Florida and New York and maintains active membership in the Florida Association of Speech-Language Pathologists and Audiologists (FLASHA), the New York State Speech-Language-Hearing Association (NYSSLHA), and the Irish Association of Speech and Language Therapists (IASLT). Her clinical experiences have traversed the lifespan, from infants to older adults, and she has also practiced clinically in schools and private practice settings. Prior to NSU, Dr. O'Connor Wells was an Instructor in the Communication Sciences Program at Hunter College, CUNY. Her primary research and clinical interests include dysphagia, aphasia in monolingual and bilingual populations, aphasia in Spanish speakers, and the aging brain. She has several journal article and book chapter publications in scholarly journals, including *Clinical Linguistics and Phonetics*, *Brain and Language*, and *Topics in Geriatric Medicine*, and has a long history of national and international conference presentations in locations such as Florida, Boston, New York, Spain, Germany, Cyprus, and Oxford University. She is currently involved in several research projects at NSU: swallowing disorders in individuals with Chagas disease in South America, viscosity of the Varibar barium product used during the modified barium swallow study, aphasia in Spanish speakers, and bilingual aphasia treatment.

Dr. Marissa Barrera is the Program Chair and Associate Professor in the graduate program in Speech-Language Pathology at Yeshiva University, New York. She received her BS in Speech-Language Pathology from Marymount Manhattan College, her MS in Speech-Language Pathology from Teacher's College, Columbia University, and her PhD in Speech-Language-Hearing Sciences from the CUNY Graduate Center. Dr. Barrera is the owner of New York Neurogenic Speech-Language Pathology, P.C., in New York City and mentors clinicians in the areas of dysphagia, motor speech, and adult cognitive-linguistic disorders.

Dr. Barrera is a recognized expert on the use of modalities (NMES, sEMG, neuromuscular taping, ultrasound) for speech and swallowing rehabilitation and provides clinical training courses globally. As a researcher and author, she has lectured in more than fifteen countries on an array of clinical topics ranging from dysphagia, NMES, motor speech disorders, cognition, and neurodegenerative diseases. She has several peer-reviewed publications and more than eighty research abstracts. She has been featured in *Women's Health*, *Vice Magazine*, *ADVANCE for Speech-Language Pathology*, and CBS News. She is a Multiple Sclerosis Certified Specialist (MSCS) and a member of the Clinical Advisory Committee of the National MS Society and the MS Foundation Advisory Board. In 2019, Dr. Barrera was awarded the Healthcare Professional Champion award from the National MS Society.

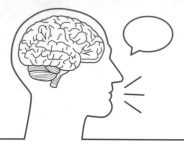

FIVE

Are We Speaking the Same Language?

Coping with Aphasia and Communication Challenges

Barbara O'Connor Wells, PhD, CCC-SLP

Linda, a retired teacher, had a stroke six months ago. Since then, she has made good progress in her twice-weekly speech therapy sessions, but she still has a long road to recovery. Speaking is very frustrating. Her words still come slowly and with lots of effort. Although she knows what she wants to say, she takes longer to come up with the words. She can sometimes get only one or two words out at a time. Occasionally, the wrong word will come out, or she will mix up the sounds in the word. She feels sad, remembering what an elegant and confident speaker she was before her stroke. Her right side is still weak, and her walking is unsteady. She now uses her left hand to write. She is thankful to have a great support system in her husband, children, and close friends. They are always patient with her when she is slow to respond and encourage her to practice what she is learning in her speech therapy sessions.

Matthew, a 75-year-old retired plumber, has been difficult to understand since he fell and experienced a brain injury last June. Although he can move his arms and legs without difficulty, his language is a big issue. He can talk, but the words he says don't always make sense to his family and friends. He doesn't say the same word the same way each time. For example, he calls his wife, Blanche, "Bladder," "Blanish," or "Blanchard" occasionally and does not seem to understand when he makes a mistake. He can't even say the name of his favorite TV show anymore: "Jeopardy" comes out as "Jello-be." It is often hard for family and friends to figure out what Matthew is trying to say.

If you are reading this chapter, you may be caring for someone with a speech-language problem caused by an acquired brain injury, degenerative disease, or other disorder. Chapter 2 covers speech problems at length. In this chapter, I discuss the concept of language. But what exactly is language?

What Is Language?

Language, in a nutshell, is the way we communicate with each other. It is an agreed-on system made up of letters or other symbols (for example, the English alphabet, Chinese characters, or the hand and facial movements of sign language). The American Speech-Language-Hearing Association (ASHA, 2021d) defines language as "the words we use and how we use them to share ideas and get what we want."

There are four "roads" to language and communication: (1) talking/speaking, (2) understanding/listening, (3) reading, and (4) writing. Our primary, or main, roads to communication are speaking and listening. Reading and writing are our secondary, or side, roads. Language is further divided into two key categories: expressive language and receptive language. Expressive language is how we express ourselves. We do this either by speaking or writing. We can also express ourselves by drawing, making gestures, or using our facial expressions. Language use can also be through technology, such as a computer or phone (for example, email or text). Receptive language is how we receive or understand communication. We do this by listening or reading. An acquired brain injury or a degenerative disease can make language and communication difficult. A person with a language disorder will have problems navigating these roads to language. This can lead to a diagnosis of aphasia.

What Is Aphasia?

You may have heard the term *aphasia* (pronounced "uh-fey-zhuh") from your loved one's medical team. Aphasia is the medical term for problems with language and communication after a stroke, acquired brain injury, brain tumor, or degenerative diseases, like dementia. Aphasia as a language disorder happens when a person has brain damage. It can make it difficult for a person to speak, understand, read, and write. It does not make a person less smart or cause problems with how they think. It is a loss of language, not intelligence (ASHA, 2021a). Brain damage can also cause other problems along with aphasia, such as speech problems (see chapter 2), swallowing problems (see chapter 4), or cognitive problems, for example, problems with memory or organizing our thoughts (see chapter 6).

How Common Is Aphasia?

According to the National Aphasia Association (2021) approximately 180,000 individuals are diagnosed with aphasia each year in the United States. It is more common for older adults to have aphasia than younger ones, although children and young adults can have an acquired brain injury, degenerative disease, or other illness that causes aphasia. The incidence of aphasia in men versus women is similar, although different aphasia types may be more common in one gender than the other. I discuss some of these different types of aphasia later in this chapter.

What Are Some Common Causes of Aphasia?

To understand what medical professionals mean by aphasia, it is important to know what medical conditions can cause language problems. Different medical issues can affect the parts of the brain responsible for language and lead to a diagnosis of aphasia.

Stroke is the most common cause of language problems and aphasia in adults. According to the National Aphasia Association (2021), about 25%–40% of individuals who survive a stroke have aphasia as one of their disabilities. A stroke may damage areas of the brain important for language, because of too much blood flow (hemorrhage) or too little blood flow (ischemia) in the brain. You may have also heard the term *brain attack*. This is a relatively new label being used in doctor's offices and public places instead of the word *stroke*. It helps the average person understand the need to get help quickly, just as in the situation of a heart attack. Important stroke symptoms that everyone should know are (1) sudden onset of slurred speech, (2) confusion, (3) weakness or numbness on one side of the body, (4) problems with vision, (5) falls, and (6) severe headaches. It is important to seek immediate medical attention if your loved one is showing signs of a stroke. You may have seen or heard about FAST. This is an acronym to help people remember the initial warning signs of a stroke. Here's what it stands for:

Face	Ask the person to smile. Does one side of the face droop?
Arm	Can the person raise both arms? Is one arm weak or numb?
Speech	Does the person sound slurred? Can they speak and understand?
Time	If you notice any of the above signs, time is of essence. Be sure to call 911 immediately to get help.

For more information on FAST, please visit the American Stroke Association (2021).

There are two main causes of stroke: hemorrhage and ischemia. Ischemia is the more common cause. In a hemorrhage, there is too much blood in or surrounding the brain, caused by a rupture, or bursting of a blood vessel, in the brain. When a brain hemorrhage occurs, oxygen may no longer be able to reach the brain areas because of the leaking or burst blood vessel. Brain cells that don't receive blood flow for more than a few minutes can die, and the functions that they control become impaired. In addition, there can be increased pressure outside or in the brain due to blood pooling. (For more information, see Cleveland Clinic, 2020).

The other cause, ischemia, is basically an opposite scenario. Here, there is a blockage in a blood vessel in the brain, which causes the area of the brain behind the blockage to not get blood. For example, if someone had atherosclerosis, where the inside of an artery narrows because of plaque buildup, a small piece of that plaque may get stuck in a blood vessel and make it hard for the blood to flow through the brain. We call this type of ischemia a *thrombosis*. If the blockage is from a blood clot that travels from somewhere else in the body to the brain, then we call it an *embolus*. For example, a piece of tumor from the lungs could break off and travel up to the brain, get lodged, and cause a blockage of blood flow. There are also mild strokes, called transient ischemic attacks (TIAs). These are also referred to as *ministrokes* and are often a warning sign that a future stroke is possible. The effects of the TIA may last only a few hours, but the warning it gives is important! It is also important to understand that people who have had one stroke are more likely to have another.

Some medical conditions cause a person to be at risk for having a stroke. These include diabetes (elevated blood sugar), hypertension (high blood pressure), obesity (abnormal fat accumulation in the body), high cholesterol, arteriosclerosis (thickening and hardening of the arteries), atrial fibrillation (heart palpitations), smoking (narrows blood vessels), and an inactive lifestyle, to name a few.

Traumatic brain injury (TBI) is another possible cause of language problems and aphasia in adults. Here, the person has had a trauma to his or her brain. The most common causes of TBI are falls and motor vehicle crashes. In the news, there has been lots of talk about sports-related TBIs, which are on the rise (for example, brain damage sustained during a football game or boxing match). There is more awareness now of this type of acquired brain injury. Some other less common causes of aphasia in adults include things like seizures (sudden and often unexpected change in brain function and consciousness), brain tumors, infections (such as meningitis), metabolic problems (such as a deficiency in vitamin B-12), or degenerative diseases or disorders, like dementia (see chapter 6). Unlike aphasia caused by stroke, in these cases, the language problems typically occur with other cognitive deficits, such as memory problems or confusion. (For more information, see Mayo Clinic, 2020.)

What Are the Areas of the Brain Responsible for Language?

To understand how language works, it is important to understand what areas of the brain are critical for language. Language is stored in and controlled by the left side of the brain in about 85% of people, whether they are right or left handed (Brookshire & McNeil, 2015). For the other 15%, language is either stored in and controlled by the right side of the brain or both sides of the brain (depending on the languages spoken).

When describing the parts of the brain, we talk about the left and right halves of the brain, called *hemispheres*. Within each half (hemisphere), there are four lobes. Each half has a frontal lobe (in the front), a temporal lobe (in the area above the ear/temple), a parietal lobe (above and behind the temporal lobe), and an occipital lobe (at the back). For the purposes of this chapter, I am highlighting the major areas of the brain where language is primarily located. The brain is a complex organ, however, and language uses many of its areas. I focus here on the two main lobes of the brain for language: the frontal and temporal lobes. (See a helpful illustration of the brain in appendix D.)

Located in the "front" part of the brain are the frontal lobes (one on the left and one on the right). The frontal lobe on the left side of the brain is important for controlling motor movements, like walking and talking. A particular part of this lobe, called *Broca's area*, is important for speaking. The frontal lobe also controls other key functions, like our attention span and personality.

The areas of the brain above our ears are called the temporal lobes. The temporal lobe in the language-dominant hemisphere (usually the left side) is important for hearing and understanding sounds. This lobe is directly behind the frontal lobe. Damage to a specific area in this lobe, called *Wernicke's area*, will lead to problems in understanding speech. The arcuate fasciculus is a band of nerve fibers that runs between Broca's and Wernicke's areas. This helps these two lobes of the brain communicate with each other.

Let's use a simple example to show how this works. Imagine that someone asks you a question (for example, "What's your name?"). Wernicke's area helps to first understand the question. To respond to the question (that is, speak), the message needs to travel to the frontal lobe of the brain. In a healthy individual, once Broca's area receives the message, the person will be able to say their response ("My name is John").

The frontal and temporal lobes of the brain both receive blood flow from the middle cerebral artery in the brain. If there is an interruption in this blood flow, then the result will be a language and communication impairment, which we call *aphasia*.

What Are Some Common Aphasia Types?

There are different types of aphasia, depending on where in the brain the damage occurs. The next section reviews the following five types: Broca's aphasia, Wernicke's aphasia, global aphasia, conduction aphasia, and anomic aphasia.

Broca's aphasia is named after Paul Broca, a famous French neurologist from the 1800s. This aphasia is sometimes called *nonfluent* or *expressive* aphasia. Broca's aphasia results from damage to the frontal lobe of the brain, where speaking is controlled. The main issue will be in expressive language. If your loved one has Broca's aphasia, they may produce single words (mostly nouns) or short phrases to communicate needs, wants, and ideas. Speech will take a lot of effort and will not have a normal rhythm to it (nonfluent). Word finding and access to words is limited in this type of aphasia. The person with Broca's aphasia may also say words different from the word they intended to say (like "vase" for "face," or "layer" for "razor") or mix up sounds in the word (like "pelsil" for "pencil"). We call these errors *paraphasias*. Persons with Broca's aphasia are often frustrated and aware of their speech and language problems and have a good understanding for things like questions and commands. So, if your loved one has this type of aphasia, they will have trouble with expressive language.

Brookshire and McNeil (2015) provide an example of speech produced by someone with Broca's aphasia using a classic picture from the Boston Diagnostic Aphasia Examination-3 called the "Cookie Theft": a kitchen scene in which a mom is washing dishes while looking out the window, and her two children are behind her, sneaking cookies from the cookie jar up high in the kitchen cabinet. In describing the picture, the person with Broca's aphasia states, "two kids . . . uh . . . stool . . . and cookie . cookie . . . jar . . . uh . . . uh . . . cabinet and stool" (2015, 194). As you can see from this example, the person has trouble finding the words to describe the picture. They use lots of filler words, such as "uh," "um," and "like" and produce one or two words at a time with lots of effort.

Persons with Broca's aphasia may be able to read simple written material, but writing is difficult. Besides the speech-language problem, those with Broca's aphasia may also have weakness on one side of the body. So, because of a left-sided stroke, the person with Broca's aphasia may also have weakness or paralysis on the right side of their body. We call this *hemiplegia* or *hemiparesis*. Because of this, the right side of their face may droop, and they may have difficulty using their right arm or leg. This can make writing difficult. The person with Broca's aphasia may have to learn to write with their other hand, and their writing will resemble how they talk. Persons with Broca's aphasia typically write in block letters and with lots of effort. What they write is usually short (single words or two- or three-word combinations) and contains just the most important words (Brookshire & McNeil, 2015).

Wernicke's aphasia is named after Carl Wernicke, a famous German physician and neurologist from the 1800s. It is sometimes called *fluent* or *receptive* aphasia. This is essentially the opposite of Broca's aphasia. These individuals don't have trouble producing words, but their words rarely make sense. They have trouble understanding the meaning of words. There is no effort in trying to talk. Their speech flows easily and with normal rhythm (fluent). Important content words, like nouns and verbs, are often missing in their speech. They may produce gibberish that you won't understand. Rate of speech and length of phrases are normal, but they have trouble with understanding. For example, if your loved one has Wernicke's aphasia, they may not understand when you ask a question or the fact that their speech does not make sense. The words they say sometimes resemble the target word (for example, "bladder" for "Blanche"), or do not resemble the desired word (for example, "sodol" for "morning"). He or she may have poor repetition skills and severely impaired reading and writing abilities. Although the person can use their hand to write, and can write with ease, the words don't make sense. They write like they speak, with no effort and with well-formed letters. But the words make little sense, and what they write lacks content (Brookshire & McNeil, 2015). A person with Wernicke's aphasia typically does not have any weakness on the opposite side of their body because the brain damage is not in the frontal lobe.

Brookshire and McNeil (2015) provide an example of speech by a person with Wernicke's aphasia. When asked to tell where he lives, the person replies, "Well, it's a meender place and it has two . . . two of them. For dreaming and pinding after supper. And up and down. Four of down and three of up" (195). This example shows the gibberish, or use of words that aren't really words or that make little sense. As you can also see from this example, it can be difficult for the listener to understand the meaning of what a person with Wernicke's aphasia is saying.

Conduction aphasia is another type of fluent aphasia. Because of damage to the arcuate fasciculus, which is a band of nerve fibers that helps Broca's and Wernicke's areas communicate, these individuals have a severe impairment in the ability to repeat, even though they can often understand the word or phrase they are asked to repeat and can otherwise say those same words or phrases fluently. They have relatively preserved language comprehension skills and are aware of the errors they make in speaking and writing. This results in frustration and attempts to correct their errors (Brookshire & McNeil, 2015). Persons with this aphasia also have anomia (word-retrieval problems) and show many paraphasias (speech errors) in spontaneous speech and repetition.

Anomic aphasia is another fluent-type aphasia. This aphasia can result from various different lesion sites in the brain (Brookshire & McNeil, 2015). Persons with this aphasia can speak fluently and with good grammar, and they can repeat, but the hallmark of their language problem is anomia (word-finding problems). They have lots of difficulty with retrieval of nouns and verbs. They are often aware and frustrated when they can't recall the word they want to say, and they may use fillers (for example, "um," "like," "that thing") or talk around the word they want to say ("You know, it's that thing you write with"). Impaired word retrieval is evident in both speech and writing.

Global aphasia is the most severe type of aphasia. This is usually the result of a large stroke that damages all the language areas of the brain. The National Institute on Deafness and Other Communication Disorders (NIDCD, 2017) states that this type of aphasia occurs when a person has extensive damage to the brain areas for language and severe difficulty with communication. In addition, these individuals cannot use reading or writing to communicate. This causes profound impairment to all roads of language. If your loved one has global aphasia, they may not talk or can say only some commonly used phrases (for example, "oh no"). The outlook for recovery in global aphasia is generally poor, and they may have long-standing problems with communication.

Unlike the above examples of nonfluent and fluent types of aphasia caused by stroke or other acquired brain injury, there is a category of aphasia called primary progressive aphasia (PPA), where an individual's language and communication skills slowly decline over time. PPA is caused by degenerative diseases, like Alzheimer's disease or frontotemporal lobar degeneration. PPA results from progressive deterioration of the areas of the brain important for speech and language. In PPA, the first symptom the individual presents with is speech and language problems, but unlike the aphasias discussed above, this type will result in progression of symptoms and decline in the ability to communicate over time. There are different types of PPA, depending on which areas of the brain are impaired at different points during the person's disease process. The three types of PPA are semantic variant of PPA (svPPA), nonfluent/agrammatic variant of PPA (nfPPA), and logopenic variant of PPA (lvPPA). The speech-language problems are initially subtle but become more severe as the brain tissue for speech and language skills continues to deteriorate. According to the National Aphasia Association (2021b), most persons with PPA will eventually end up mute (unable to talk) and will be unable to understand what they hear or read. Although the first symptoms are problems with speech and language, other problems associated with degenerative disease, such as memory loss or behavior changes, will surface later. For more information on PPA, see the National Aphasia Association (2021a) and chapter 6.

What Does Recovery Look Like?

The National Aphasia Association (2021b) reminds us that there is no cure for aphasia. A big part of the mystery is that no two brains are alike, so we cannot give definite answers about a particular person's recovery. The doctor, speech-language pathologist (SLP), and other medical professionals will consider multiple factors when creating a *prognosis for recovery*. This means how likely your loved one is to recover language over time and with speech therapy. Although we cannot predict the future and whether your loved one will improve, there are certain positive and negative signs for recovery. It is important to know that if the aphasia lasts more than the first few months after a stroke or other acquired brain injury, a complete recovery is not likely to occur. On a positive note, however, a person with aphasia may continue to recover, even ten or more years later. As the caregiver, it is important to your loved one's recovery that you continue with the recommended speech treatment and help they stay motivated and positive throughout the process of recovery. And if your loved one is diagnosed with PPA, it is critical to be there to support them as their communication skills worsen over time.

What Are Some Factors That Can Influence Recovery?

Severity of deficits: A person who suffers a mild stroke or TBI will likely recover better than someone who had a severe stroke or TBI.

Age: A person young at the time of their stroke or other medical cause of aphasia will probably have better recovery than someone who is older. For example, a person who has a stroke in their fifties will probably recover better than someone in their eighties.

First-time stroke or brain injury: If this is your loved one's first and only stroke or brain injury, they have a better chance of recovery than if this is the third or fourth stroke or injury.

New stroke or brain injury: Someone who recently had a stroke or brain injury may show gradual or even quick recovery in the first few weeks or months compared to someone who had their stroke or brain injury a few years ago.

Overall health: Someone who is otherwise healthy will recover better than someone who is frail and has many medical complications.

Motivation: Good motivation and a positive support system will help in your loved one's recovery.

Education level: Someone with a higher level of education (for example, college and beyond) may have stimulated their brain over time more than someone with less education.

Language status: Research has shown that a bilingual speaker or speaker of three or more languages uses more brain resources to speak. Therefore, speaking more than one language can help individuals with aphasia recover their language skills better than those who speak only one language. (For more information, see Brain Facts, 2008.)

How Is Aphasia Evaluated?

If the medical team suspects a person has aphasia, they will send a referral to a licensed SLP for an evaluation. One of the key medical professionals who evaluates and recommends a person with a stroke for rehabilitation is the neurologist. A neurologist is a medical doctor who specializes in diagnosing, treating, and managing disorders of the brain and nervous system, such as stroke, TBI, Parkinson's disease, and amyotrophic lateral sclerosis. The neurologist will do a thorough workup of your loved one's neurological system, including the various nerves that run through the body and how they communicate with the brain and muscles. Another important member of the medical team is the physiatrist. This is a medical doctor who has expertise in rehabilitation medicine. The physiatrist will often oversee the rehabilitation process and communicate closely with the other team members, such as the physical therapist (PT), occupational therapist (OT), SLP, and you, the caregiver.

The SLP will be the team member with experience and expertise in evaluating and diagnosing aphasia. They will use lots of different tools to test your loved one's language, to determine communication strengths and weaknesses. There are both informal and formal ways to assess language, and a thorough evaluation of language includes both types of evaluation.

Informal Evaluation

The SLP may use everyday materials in the hospital room or in your loved one's home to examine language. If your loved one is in the hospital, the SLP might select objects in their room, such as a toothbrush, pen, and cup, and use them as part of the evaluation. A typical assessment starts with open-ended questions, such as "How are you?" or "What happened to you?" This is an important part of the assessment, because the SLP is looking to see how well your loved one can take part in conversation. The SLP will look for things such as whether your loved one produces words or sentences, how long the sentences are, if the words or sentences answer the question, and how clear and smooth the speech is. Also, the SLP wants to find out how much your loved one remembers about what happened to them.

For receptive language, the SLP may ask your loved one to follow some directions (such as "shake your head," or "touch your nose"); identify things like body parts, colors, everyday objects (such as "cup"); read words and match them to the object; and read a sentence and select the written answer, to name a few.

For expressive language, the SLP may ask your loved one to repeat words, phrases, and sentences; name common objects; name items in a category (such as "name all the fruits you can think of in one minute"); answer yes or no and wh- questions ("Are you John?" "Where do you live?"); write letters of the alphabet; write their name; copy letters or numbers; and write a sentence that the SLP says or write a sentence independently.

Because cognition (which includes skills like attention, memory, and problem solving) is so closely partnered with language, the SLP will want to test this area. This may include seeing how alert and responsive your loved one is, how attentive they are, and how strong their memory is. This may include such things as asking where they were born, what their children's names are (long-term memory), what they had for breakfast (short-term memory), and whether they can repeat a list of numbers (immediate memory).

Formal Evaluation

It is beyond the scope of this book to describe all the formal tests available to evaluate language problems in adults. Nonetheless, it is worth mentioning the names of a few, so you might become familiar with them. These would include the Boston Diagnostic Aphasia Examination-3, the Boston Naming Test-2, and the Western Aphasia Battery-Revised. The SLP will decide which tests are most appropriate to give your loved one to evaluate their language strengths and weaknesses. Sometimes, the SLP will include other types of tests in a comprehensive evaluation, such as tests to evaluate memory and cognition (for example, Ross Information Processing Assessment-2).

How Is Aphasia Treated?

As with formal tests, it is beyond this chapter to list all the treatment programs and approaches to help improve language skills in someone with aphasia. It is important for you, the caregiver, however, to be aware of the general areas that an SLP may work on to improve language. Treatment for aphasia should always be individualized to the specific problem areas identified during the evaluation. There are many ways to work on improving your loved one's language. The treatment they get will depend on many factors, including you and your loved one's goals for therapy, motivation, how severe the impairment is, and areas of language affected. Your loved one may work with an SLP on their own, or in a small group. Family involvement is an important part of treatment, so that goals and activities can continue at home. Your loved one's SLP may also suggest a local aphasia support group to promote socialization. Ultimately, treatment should help them meet their highest level of function and ability to take part in daily activities. Treatment should aim to either restore impaired functions or compensate for residual deficits.

A current direction in aphasia treatment is collaboration between the patient, their families, and the SLP. We call this Person- and Family-Centered Care. In this model of treatment, the person with aphasia and their family are stakeholders and equal partners in the therapy process. Therapy goals incorporate the needs and preferences of the person with aphasia and their family. The SLP and other rehabilitation team members wear multiple hats in this approach to treatment, including therapist, counselor, cheerleader, and advocate for the person with aphasia. For more information on Person- and Family-Centered Care, see ASHA (2021b).

Treatment for Receptive Language Problems

When an SLP is targeting receptive language skills in treatment, the overall goal is to improve comprehension, or understanding. The goals set should be reasonable for your loved one to work toward, based on the severity of their language problem. For severe receptive language problems, the SLP may work at the word level. Things like understanding sentences and conversation are way too difficult at this point. For example, the SLP may have your loved one select a common object by name when given two choices (for example, cup vs. spoon), opposite concepts (up vs. down), and simple one-word directions ("smile"). If your loved one's deficits are less severe and they can understand at the sentence level, tasks may include answering yes or no questions ("Is your name Bob?"), following simple directions ("point to your nose"), or selecting a picture that matches the spoken sentence ("Which one shows the girl is eating"). For mild deficits, where your loved one can participate in conversation, therapy activities may include things like listening to a story and answering questions about it, or answering open-ended questions ("Tell me about your best friend").

In the home, you can easily work on improving receptive language skills during your daily activities. For example, include your loved one in meal preparation. Ask them to select, point to, or hand you specific ingredients by name (for example, butter), follow directions ("Pass me the salt"), or remember a series of directions ("What was the first thing we needed to do?"). When watching a TV show together, you can ask follow-up questions to check for comprehension (for example, "Where does the show take place?" "What is the main character's name?").

The other component of receptive language is reading comprehension. For someone with severe aphasia, the lowest level of reading would be "survival" reading. This would be making sure your loved one can read word-level signs, like "STOP" or "Danger." Beyond that, at the single-word level, the SLP may work on having your loved one select a written word when given a choice of two words or match a written name of the object with the object itself or a picture of the object. The focus would be everyday vocabulary items, such as common items around the house. The vocabulary items can even be in themes (for example, vocabulary associated with the kitchen, like fork, spoon, cup, oven). At the single-word level, the SLP may work on having your loved one select a written word when the other choice is similar (for example, cat vs. hat). The SLP can also work on reading by having your loved one select the missing letter(s) in a target word. At a higher level, as your loved one understands sentences and longer reading material, this may involve things like selecting the written word that completes the sentence (open the door vs. cup; bake the cookies in the oven vs. in the fridge). At the sentence level, goals for reading can also involve rearranging the words in a sentence (sentence scramble) or matching a picture with the target written sentence. Higher-level reading activities might involve functional reading skills, like reading the labels on medications, reading and following the written instructions of a recipe, or reading sections of a favorite book or newspaper and answering questions to show understanding.

Treatment for Expressive Language Problems

The SLP will again keep in mind your loved one's ability level and the severity of their deficits in expressive language to create treatment goals. The overall goal will be to use any or all forms of expression for communication. This may be speaking, writing, augmentative alternative systems (for example, picture symbols or computerized devices), or gestures for communication (see chapter 2 for more information). For severe deficits, the SLP may work on getting your loved one to produce often used speech. This can include activities such as counting 1 to 10, reciting the alphabet, and labeling or naming simple pictures. When your loved one is having trouble naming a common object, you can help them by providing the first sound or first syllable of the word, putting the word in a carrier phrase, providing a rhyming word, telling your loved one what the object is used for (function), or where the object is typically kept (location). These are some helpful cues for word finding.

Sentence completion is another helpful activity. This is where you provide the start of a sentence and ask your loved one to finish it (for example, "open the —— "). Later, you can make the sentences more open ended and less specific, where there might be different words that can fill in the end of the sentence (for example, "In the summer we like to —— "). Repetition is another important area of expressive language. This is where you ask your loved one to repeat simple words (for example, "dog"), then short phrases ("I'm hungry"), and then longer sentences ("In the morning, I drink coffee"). If your loved one has milder deficits in expressive language, you can use story elaboration. This happens when you start a short story and ask them, "What do you think will happen next?" Your loved one may also benefit from picture description tasks, where you present a busy picture and ask them to describe what is going on. Procedural discourse is another great strategy that your loved one's SLP may use in therapy. The SLP would ask your loved one to describe how to do a common task (for example, "Tell me how you make a cup of coffee").

Another important road for expression is writing. In therapy, your loved one can practice writing the alphabet, their name and address, the names of common objects, sentences about everyday routines, a description of a busy picture, or other functional writing tasks, like learning how to write grocery lists, filling out checks to pay household bills, and so on.

In severe cases, your loved one may need to find other ways to express themselves. These may include simple hand gestures; sign language; a picture board with everyday needs and wants; phrase boards if your loved one can understand phrases; alphabet boards, for individuals who have functional spelling skills (for an example, see appendix B); computerized systems, such as a dedicated augmentative/alternative communication (AAC) device; or even apps for a tablet or smartphone. The person with aphasia can use AAC devices as self-cueing strategies. For example, if your loved one has trouble coming up with the word they want to say, an alphabet board can help him or her give you, the listener, the first letter of that word. Your loved one's SLP will determine if they need an AAC system to communicate better. It is important that you, the caregiver, are an active part of the training on the AAC system, so they can use the device outside the therapy room.

The American Speech-Language-Hearing Association (2021a) has a helpful document that outlines all the different approaches to aphasia therapy. Some approaches are aimed at helping the person with aphasia take part, to the fullest extent possible, in their community. Group therapy for aphasia is one such approach. In group treatment, the members with aphasia can engage in functional activities that incorporate their previous hobbies and interests, such as playing Bingo, Jeopardy!, music trivia, and meal preparation. Group therapy is a great outlet of support for both persons with aphasia and their caregivers.

Another community-based approach to aphasia therapy is Life Participation Approach to Aphasia (LPAA). In this approach, the focus is on what the person can do and how to get them back to tak-

ing part in daily activities, rather than focusing on remediating specific problem areas. This approach engages the person with aphasia
outside the therapy room, with activities at home and in the community. The goal is to help improve the quality of life of the person with
aphasia by creating therapy goals that produce meaningful real-life
outcomes. For example, the person with aphasia may want to give a
speech at their daughter's upcoming wedding or order their favorite
coffee at Starbucks. In collaboration with the SLP, the person with
aphasia and their family would work on functional and patient-driven
therapy goals.

Other approaches include computer-based therapy (for example, apps and other software programs on a computer, tablet, or
smartphone that can target language goals). Some of these programs
even collect information to track progress, which can be included
in documentation to support continued therapy. Another approach
is Melodic Intonation Therapy (MIT), which is based on the idea
that the unimpaired right side of the brain, which is used to appreciate music, melody, and rhythm, can help with speech output on
the impaired left side of the brain. The person learns to "sing" target
words and phrases, using a simple up and down intonation. As the
person improves, they come to rely less and less on "singing" to produce speech.

Other programs use picture symbols to help improve communication skills (for example, Promoting Aphasics' Communication
Effectiveness, or PACE), while others teach persons with aphasia how
to use gestures to communicate (for example, Visual Action Therapy,
or VAT). Still others focus on improving word retrieval. A popular
approach to word retrieval is Semantic Feature Analysis (SFA) treatment, where the person learns to use the specific features of a target
object to help recall its name. For example, if the target vocabulary
word is *cup*, the person with aphasia would use the SFA chart to talk

about the features of a cup (for example, what it's used for, where you find it, what other objects are like it).

An important question posed by some loved ones is whether a person with aphasia can return to work. This can be a concern, especially for a younger stroke survivor who is the breadwinner for the family. Sometimes, a person with aphasia can eventually return to work, but there are a lot of factors to consider, such as how severe the impairment is, age, motivation, family supports, and type of employment. If you and your loved one have concerns about returning to work and want to incorporate work-related skills into therapy, be sure to address that with your loved one's medical team.

What If My Loved One Speaks More Than One Language?

Does your loved one speak more than one language? They may speak and understand better in one language than the other. Or your loved one may have trouble speaking and understanding in all their languages. If they spoke more than one language before their stroke, it is important to make sure the SLP is aware of that. When evaluating a person with aphasia who speaks more than one language, it is important to think about the languages they spoke, the age(s) when they learned the languages, the order in which the languages were learned, the use of the languages before the aphasia, and which language or languages are most needed to return to daily activities. Ideally, the SLP will evaluate all the languages your loved one spoke and include all of them in the speech therapy treatment goals. One common tool to evaluate the languages of a bilingual speaker is the Bilingual Aphasia Test (BAT). This test, developed by Michel Paradis and colleagues at McGill University, is an evaluation tool designed to test the language skills of all the languages spoken by a bilingual speaker. It is currently available in seventy-four different languages, from Amharic to Yiddish. Each test is equivalent across the different languages and is not a mere translation from one language to another. For more information, see McGill University Department of Linguistics (2021).

If it is not possible to test and treat all the previously spoken languages in therapy, we recommend that your loved one continue to be exposed to the other languages they spoke, as much as possible. You can do this, for example, by watching TV and listening to radio in the other languages, going to a favorite Spanish or French restaurant, or continuing to have friends and family speak the other languages to them.

Which language comes back first and best after a stroke, brain injury, or other neurological disease or disorder? For some bilingual speakers, the language the person spoke first will be the first and best one to recover. This would be their native language. For others, it's the language they used the most (which can also be their first, or native, language). And for some, it's the language they have the most emotional ties with. The most common recovery pattern, however, is *parallel recovery*, when the two or more languages the person speaks recover at the same time. See Ardila and Ramos (2007) and Paradis (2004) for more detail on this topic of bilingualism and bilingual aphasia. Boston University's Aphasia Research Laboratory also has information on some current projects on bilingual aphasia treatment.

What Happens When the Right Side of the Brain Is Damaged?

When the brain damage is to the right side of the brain instead of the left side, this can lead to different symptoms that affect language and communication. Some common features of right brain damage include changes in personality, rambling speech that goes off topic, problems with understanding the meaning of expressions like "don't cry over spilled milk," and poor attention and focus. These individuals may also have problems with vision and body awareness of the left side, which can lead to safety issues. They may bump into things on the left side or have trouble reading words on the left side of a page. They may even not recognize their own left side. I remember a young man with brain injury who would ask me almost every therapy session, "Where's my left arm?" It was numb, and he could not feel it, and he could not see on his left side. I would have to raise it up for him to see, and then he would give a sigh of relief and continue with our therapy activities.

Individuals with right brain damage may also have difficulty with reading and writing, and when asked to draw a clock, they may leave off the left side of it or scrunch all the numbers on the right side. The person may be impulsive and not think about the consequences of their actions. Individuals with right brain damage may appear emotionless and almost robotic. They may have difficulty recognizing other people's emotions (for example, they may miss that someone's voice sounds shaky because they are upset). When the person writes or speaks, the words come easily, but they make little sense and don't really speak to the topic at hand. They may even have trouble recognizing familiar faces. When they talk, they ramble and don't allow the conversation partner a chance to talk. They may no longer understand jokes and may not laugh at the punch lines. In addition, persons with right brain damage often do not realize the extent of their deficits, and they may be unmotivated for therapy as a result (Brookshire & McNeil, 2015).

When I was an SLP working in a medical setting, I evaluated a woman who had a right-side brain stroke. When I got to her room, she was sitting on the right side of the bed, grooming herself. As I approached her from her left side and called her name, she had no reaction. When I came into her view and she could see me with the right side of her eyes, she smiled and said hello. Despite having a mirror in front of her, I was shocked to see how she had groomed herself. On the right side, her hair and makeup were perfect. On her left side, however, her hair was disheveled, and her makeup was all over the place. Her lipstick was halfway up her cheek. She had glasses on, but the lens on the left side was broken, and the glasses were hanging crookedly on her nose. Her speech was rambling and off topic. I had trouble getting her to let me speak so I could ask her the questions I needed to test her speech. When I asked her what "don't cry over spilled milk" meant, she looked at the floor for spilled milk and told me I should clean it up.

How Is Right-Side Brain Damage Treated?

Although less is known about the treatment outcomes for the communication problems seen in individuals with right-brain damage than for persons with aphasia, these individuals require access to treatment as much as people with aphasia due to left-side brain damage (Hewetson, Cornwell, & Shum, 2017). Treatment for communication problems due to right-brain damage focuses on addressing behavioral and cognitive areas that impact communication. For behavioral issues, like impulsivity, or what we perceive as rude behavior, some effective strategies include providing specific feedback about inappropriate behaviors. For example, you might point out that laughing is not the appropriate response to bad news, or that it was not their turn to speak. The hope and expectation over time is that your loved one with right-brain damage will monitor their own behaviors. For poor attention and distractible behaviors, the SLP may use activities to target better focus. For example, there are computer activities that can help improve attention. Listening to a story in background noise can challenge your loved one's attention span. If they enjoy things like crossword puzzles or Sudoku, these would be helpful and fun ways to target paying attention. For impulsivity, the SLP may teach you to put "stop and go" signals around the house. The big issue with impulsivity is that it can make things like walking and eating dangerous (for example, your loved one may try to get up out of bed without help or stuff too much food into their mouth without paying attention during meals). For difficulty with problem solving, the SLP may work with picture cards that show a problem situation and see if your loved one can identify the problem (for example, a picture of a house on fire—"What's the problem?"), as well as working on problem solving in real-world situations (for example, in the kitchen). For left-sided visual neglect, the SLP may work on improving your loved one's awareness of their left side by sitting on their left side and putting items on that side, to force them to look left. In reading tasks, you can highlight the left border of the page in yellow and teach your loved one to "look for the yellow" when reading. This will ensure that they are not missing crucial words when reading. ASHA (2021c) provides additional helpful information on right brain damage and communication.

What Are Some Tips for Better Communication with My Loved One with Language and Communication Problems?

Many helpful websites related to aphasia have tips for better communication with your loved one with a language problem (see the list of resources at the end of this chapter). The following are some common tips for better communication with your loved one with a language and communication problem:

> **Attention:** Get your loved one's attention first by calling their name. Be sure they are ready to take part in conversation with you.

Eye contact: Keep eye contact with your loved one throughout the communication exchange. Eye contact will help you know if your loved one is paying attention, understands you, or is confused. Your loved one can also get helpful information from your facial expressions and body language as you talk with them (for example, watching your mouth as you speak, seeing you smile or frown to show emotion, or watching your hand movements).

Environment: Communicate in an optimum environment. Make sure the environment is free of distractions. Turn off the TV or radio. Turn on the lights and make sure the environment is well lit and that you are standing close enough for your loved one to see your mouth and hear you.

Keep your words short and simple but adult: Make sure you are not "talking down" to your loved one. Repeat any keywords important for your loved one to understand. And don't shout, unless your loved one is hard of hearing.

Speak slowly: Slow your speech and allow your loved one time to understand what you said.

Use yes or no questions as appropriate: Yes or no questions are easier to understand and answer than ones for which your loved one needs to come up with their own answer.

Find other ways to communicate: If your loved one does not understand you, use other ways to communicate. For example, you can try using drawings, gestures, pointing, writing, and facial expressions to help your loved one better understand. You can also have your loved one try one or more alternate ways to communicate when they are having trouble talking. The Aphasia Institute outlines some of these alternate ways as tools to support your loved one in conversation. In supported conversation, the conversation partner (that's you!) can use a variety of tools to help improve the information exchange between you and your loved one with aphasia. To help with information exchange (that is, understanding: getting the information "in"; and response: getting the information "out") the caregiver needs to know that not all communication involves speaking and listening.

Anticipate your loved one's needs, wants, and ideas: Try to figure out what your loved one might attempt to communicate in specific situations. For example, if you know there's specific vocabulary that surrounds breakfast each day, and a select list of things your loved one likes to have for breakfast, then try to predict what they might want to have for breakfast. If they are struggling to say a word that begins with j, then maybe offer, "Do you want juice?" Knowing your loved one's daily routine will help you figure out their daily needs, wants, and ideas.

Be a good listener: Listen intently and ask your loved one to repeat if needed. You may also rephrase the question for them (for example, "I think you are asking for more coffee —is that right?").

Be patient: Be as patient as possible and don't rush the communication exchange between you and your loved one. It may take longer than usual.

Mistakes are okay: Your loved one may continue to make mistakes, such as choosing the wrong word or sounds to communicate. Give them a chance to speak and repair the communication as much as possible. Praise when communication attempts are successful and try not to dwell on mistakes made.

Offer help: Try not to answer for or finish your loved one's sentences. If they are struggling or stuck on a word, offer help and respect if your loved one does not want help at that moment.

Additionally, be sure to include your loved one in important decision making for them and the family. You may need to set up a system for your loved one to communicate their thoughts, such as a yes/no board or an alphabet board (see appendix B). I remember an older lady unable to speak as a result of a stroke. Her family spoke to the medical team members in front of her and made medical decisions for her without including her in those important decisions. One day, when I went to see her and put her alphabet board in front of her, she used it to tell me she did not want to be DNR (Do Not Resuscitate).

What Are the Important Take-Home Points in This Chapter?

- Aphasia is the medical term for language and communication problems caused by neurological issues, such as a stroke.

- There are different types of aphasia, with different problems that impact speaking, listening, reading, and writing. The areas in the brain that are damaged will determine what type of aphasia your loved one may have.

- There are various factors that can affect how a person recovers their language skills, such as age, severity of deficits, motivation, and family support.

- If the medical team suspects language and communication problems, the SLP will be the expert on the team and work closely with other professionals to diagnose and treat aphasia.

- Language and communication problems can be improved or compensated for by speech-language therapy, conducted by an SLP.

- There are many helpful tips for how best to communicate with your loved one with aphasia, such as speaking slowly and being a good listener.

In conclusion, the goal of this chapter is to inform you, the caregiver, about language and communication problems your loved one may experience after acquired brain injury or degenerative disease. I hope you have found this information useful and that it will help you and your loved one "speak the same language" again.

REFERENCES

American Speech-Language-Hearing Association (ASHA). (2021a). *Aphasia.* Retrieved February 2, 2021. https://www.asha.org/public/speech/disorders/Aphasia/.

American Speech-Language-Hearing Association (ASHA). (2021b). *Person- and family-centered care.* Retrieved February 2, 2021. https://www.asha.org/Practice-Portal/Clinical-Topics/Aphasia/Person-and-Family-Centered-Care/.

American Speech-Language-Hearing Association (ASHA). (2021c). *Right hemisphere damage.* Retrieved February 2, 2021. https://www.asha.org/practice-portal/clinical-topics/right-hemisphere-damage/.

American Speech-Language-Hearing Association (ASHA). (2021d). *What is speech? What is language?* Retrieved February 2, 2021. https://www.asha.org/public/speech/development/speech-and-language/.

American Stroke Association. (2021). *F.A.S.T Infographic.* Retrieved March 1,

2021. https://www.stroke.org/en/help-and-support/resource-library
/fast-materials/2019-fast-infographic.

Ardila, A., & Ramos, E. (Eds.). (2007). *Speech and language disorders in bilinguals.* Nova Science.

Brain Facts. (2008, September 1). *The bilingual brain.* https://www.brainfacts
.org/Archives/2008/The-Bilingual-Brain.

Brookshire, R. H., & McNeil, M. R. (2015). *Introduction to neurogenic communication disorders* (8th ed.). Mosby Elsevier.

Cleveland Clinic. (2020, May 4). *Brain bleed, hemorrhage (intracranial hemorrhage).* https://my.clevelandclinic.org/health/diseases/14480-brain-bleed
-hemorrhage-intracranial-hemorrhage.

Hewetson, R., Cornwell, P., & Shum, D. (2017). Cognitive-communication disorder following right hemisphere stroke: Exploring rehabilitation access and outcomes. *Topics in Stroke Rehabilitation, 24*(5), 330–36.

Mayo Clinic. (2020, October 20). *Aphasia.* https://www.mayoclinic.org
/diseases-conditions/aphasia/symptoms-causes/syc-20369518.

McGill University Department of Linguistics. (2021). *Bilingual aphasia test (BAT).* Retrieved February 2, 2021. https://www.mcgill.ca/linguistics
/research/bat.

National Aphasia Association. (2021a). *Aphasia definitions.* Retrieved February 2, 2021. https://www.aphasia.org/aphasia-definitions/.

National Aphasia Association. (2021b). *Aphasia FAQs.* Retrieved February 2, 2021. http://www.aphasia.org/aphasia-faqs/.

National Institute on Deafness and Other Communication Disorders. (2017, March 6). *Aphasia.* https://www.nidcd.nih.gov/health/aphasia.

Paradis, M. (2004). *A neurolinguistic theory of bilingualism.* Benjamins.

RESOURCES

Adler Aphasia Center: https://adleraphasiacenter.org/
American Heart Association: https://www.heart.org/
American Speech-Language-Hearing Association: https://www.asha.org
American Stroke Association: https://www.stroke.org/
American Stroke Foundation: https://americanstroke.org/

Aphasia Access: Life Participation Approach to Aphasia (LPAA): https://www
.aphasiaaccess.org

The Aphasia Center: https://theaphasiacenter.com/

Aphasia Institute: https://www.aphasia.ca/

Aphasia Research Laboratory at Boston University: https://www.bu.edu
/aphasiaresearch/

Brain Injury Association of America: https://www.biausa.org/

Cleveland Clinic: https://my.clevelandclinic.org

Mayo Clinic: https://www.mayoclinic.org

National Aphasia Association: https://www.aphasia.org/

Voices of Hope for Aphasia: http://www.vohaphasia.org/

ABOUT THE AUTHOR

Dr. Barbara O'Connor Wells is an Associate Professor and Clinical Supervisor
in the Department of Speech-Language Pathology at Nova Southeastern University (NSU). She received her BA in Speech Pathology and Audiology and her
MA in Speech-Language Pathology from St. John's University, New York, and
her PhD in Speech-Language-Hearing Sciences from the Graduate Center of
the City University of New York (CUNY). She teaches coursework and supervises individual and group treatment sessions in the areas of dysphagia, motor
speech, and adult language disorders at NSU.

Dr. O'Connor Wells is certified by the American Speech-Language-Hearing Association (ASHA) and has twenty-five years of experience in acute, subacute, long-term, and homecare rehabilitation of adult neurogenic communication, cognition, and swallowing disorders. She is licensed in both Florida
and New York and maintains active membership in the Florida Association of
Speech-Language Pathologists and Audiologists (FLASHA), the New York State
Speech-Language-Hearing Association (NYSSLHA), and the Irish Association
of Speech and Language Therapists (IASLT). Her clinical experiences have traversed the lifespan, from infants to older adults, and she has also practiced clinically in schools and private practice settings. Prior to NSU, Dr. O'Connor Wells
was an Instructor in the Communication Sciences Program at Hunter College,
CUNY. Her primary research and clinical interests include dysphagia, aphasia

in monolingual and bilingual populations, aphasia in Spanish speakers, and the aging brain. She has several journal article and book chapter publications in scholarly journals, including *Clinical Linguistics and Phonetics*, *Brain and Language*, and *Topics in Geriatric Medicine*, and has a long history of national and international conference presentations in locations such as Florida, Boston, New York, Spain, Germany, Cyprus, and Oxford University. She is currently involved in several research projects at NSU: swallowing disorders in individuals with Chagas disease in South America, viscosity of the Varibar barium product used during the modified barium swallow study, aphasia in Spanish speakers, and bilingual aphasia treatment.

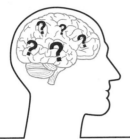

SIX

Another Senior Moment, or Is It Something Else?

Communicating with Those Who Have Dementia

Elizabeth Roberts, PhD, CCC-SLP

Cassandra is a 55-year-old wife and mother of three with a high-stress position as a corporate financial officer, a job that frequently requires 10- to 12-hour workdays. As she enters her home after a long day's work to the sounds of the family in the den, she rushes to put away her keys without thinking about it. Her attention is now focused on preparation of the meal she has planned for a family that includes three growing teenage boys. The next morning, she prepares herself to rush out the door. She begins a frantic search for those keys, eventually finding them in the pocket of her coat, instead of on the hook by the front door.

Cassandra is experiencing what we may call "a senior moment." Her attention was diverted from her keys to her kids just as she was putting the keys away. Stress is a known factor in the development of people's frequent inability to attend to their actions (Petrac et al., 2009). The ability to pay attention to more than one task or item at the same time, known as divided attention, may be especially compromised. Cassandra has a stress-provoking lifestyle in this period of her life, and she may continue to exhibit signs of age-associated memory impairment until she learns to use strategies to control her stress. An example of this compensation would be to train herself to put the keys on the same hook each time she enters her home. This action will eventually become habitual and will no longer require her attention as she puts her keys away in that designated spot without even thinking about it.

Max is a 66-year-old man who recently retired from his job and is adjusting to a new life of freedom and, unfortunately, long periods of inactivity with few social interactions. Max has a history of alcoholism that began in his early thirties, when he filled his days with two-martini lunches with coworkers and then three or more drinks most evenings at home for dinnertime or at the local pub. As the years progressed, his consumption increased, and he began to display lapses in his memory, even when not under the influence of alcohol. While he recently joined Alcoholics Anonymous to curtail his drinking and to save his relationships, the damage to his brain has already advanced. He has shown no improvement in the memory lapses he has been experiencing, and his bouts of irritability continue to disrupt his life and the lives of others.

Max is exhibiting signs of alcohol-related dementia long after finally becoming sober. Signs of this type of dementia in his behavior include acting inappropriately in public or lashing out with sudden outbursts of anger. He now lives alone after his wife divorced him five years ago, and his home is unkempt, as is his physical appearance. He has also been neglecting his financial obligations because of his problems with planning and organization. He has few friends at this point. His apparent lack of compassion or understanding of the feelings of others has caused many to avoid him. Because of his alcohol-related dementia, he may eventually end up in a nursing home because his personality issues and inability to care for himself will progress and place him in ever-increasing danger.

———

If you are reading this chapter, you may be caring for a loved one who has dementia. The hope is that this chapter will help guide you in caring for and enriching your communication with your loved one. Many people in middle age or older have experienced what we commonly call "a senior moment," like *Cassandra* in the first case study. A quick trip to retrieve a glass of water results in the person standing in the kitchen and wondering why they are there. Upon meeting for lunch, a person may suddenly not be able to remember a lifelong friend's name. They may attempt to mask this sudden, surprising lapse of memory while a wave of concern comes across their mind. Is this another senior moment, or is it something else? These types of events may cause people to wonder if they are experiencing early signs of dementia. These senior moments are common in middle age, and even young people have lapses in memory. They could be a cause for concern or simply a sign of age-associated memory impairment, a benign condition frequently observed as we age, as discussed in chapter 1. Or these lapses in memory can be an early sign of something else. Let's begin with mild cognitive impairment, which might be the first concerning sign of memory decline that eventually leads to dementia.

What Is Mild Cognitive Impairment?

Mild cognitive impairment (MCI) is a classification of cognitive or memory decline that was first used as a clinical diagnosis in the 1980s. In 2013, the American Psychiatric Association (APA) changed the classification in the 5th edition of the *Diagnostic and Statistical Manual of Mental Disorders (DSM-5)* to "mild neurocognitive disorder." Criteria for mild neurocognitive disorder are identified as "evidence of modest cognitive decline from a previous level in one or more cognitive domains: complex attention, executive function, learning and memory, perceptual-motor, and social cognition" (APA, 2013).

A neurologist makes this diagnosis based on information provided by the individual, a knowledgeable informant such as family member, or a clinician or health care worker, any of whom are concerned that this individual is experiencing some type of cognitive decline or difficulties remembering. This diagnosis should be confirmed by a standardized neuropsychological test. In addition, the APA (2013) suggests that for MCI to be the diagnosis, these deficits should not interfere with a person's independence and performance of activities of daily living (ADLs). These cognitive problems must occur outside episodes of delirium (temporary confusion and disorientation) and not be a sign of another mental disorder. According to the *DSM-5*, mild neurocognitive disorder can precede major neurocognitive disorder, more commonly referred to as *dementia*.

Not all persons who experience mild neurocognitive disorder will experience further cognitive deterioration into dementia (APA, 2013). Progression rates vary among individuals. A thorough medical examination is required to identify these early changes and provide information regarding the possible progression into dementia. The next section describes some of the more common forms of dementia.

What Is Dementia and What Are Some Common Types?

Medical professionals who have the expertise to diagnose major neurocognitive disorder, or dementia, are typically neurologists. Geriatric psychiatrists, neuropsychologists, and geriatricians may also be qualified to diagnose this condition. While the APA acknowledges that use of the word *dementia* will persist, they agreed to no longer use the term in their manual to avoid the stigma associated with this word. *Dementia* comes from a Latin term for "mad" or "insane." This disorder is progressive and debilitating and can cause multiple impairments; however, madness or insanity are absolutely not among them. Despite the change in the use of the word by the APA, dementia is still the prevalent term used to represent this disorder. For example, the Alzheimer's Association continues to use the term dementia rather than major neurocognitive disorder.

Impairments associated with dementia are problems with short-term memory, long-term memory, abstract thinking, judgment, and language as well as other symptoms specific to certain types of this disorder. These impairments are severe enough to interfere with the person's ability to work, socialize, and perform daily tasks, such as washing dishes, making beds, and preparing meals. Persons with dementia may frequently forget the names of their loved ones and look disheveled in appearance, in how they keep their homes, and in how they tend to their financial affairs.

While many people assume Alzheimer's disease and dementia are the same, this is not the case. Alzheimer's dementia is only one type of dementia. The word *dementia* is a broad term for this cognitive disorder, and there are different forms of it. While Alzheimer's disease dementia is the most common type, accounting for approximately 60%–80% of all cases, there are many others (Alzheimer's Association, 2021a–c). Included in these are vascular dementia, Parkinson's dementia, frontotemporal dementia, and alcohol-related dementia. These all have different signs and symptoms and differences in how they progress. Keep in mind, too, that more than one type of dementia may be present in the same person. For example, a person with Alzheimer's disease may also develop dementia caused by a stroke or secondary to Parkinson's disease. In the next sections of this chapter, I describe the main types of dementia. Johns Hopkins University Press publishes a book entitled *Is It Alzheimer's?: 101 Answers to Your Most Pressing Questions about Memory Loss and Dementia*, which provides an excellent overview on this topic.

Alzheimer's Disease Dementia

Alzheimer's disease (AD) dementia is the most common form. According to APA (2013), AD is among the major neurocognitive disorders (major NCDs) that cause problems in six major cognitive areas: (1) complex attention, which includes sustained attention, divided attention, selective attention, and information-processing speed; (2) executive function, which includes planning, decision making, working memory, and mental flexibility (the person's ability to switch from one activity or topic to another); (3) learning and memory, which include recall, recognition, and other facets of memory; (4) language, which includes word finding, grammar and syntax, and understanding language; (5) perceptual-motor function, which includes visual perception; and (6) social cognition, which includes recognition of emotions and insight. To be diagnosed with a major NCD, there must be evidence of significant decline in one or more of these domains.

For a diagnosis of major NCD due to AD, there must be problems with memory, thinking, judgment, and reasoning that impairs a person's ability to function in their daily life. The deteriorating nature of this disease will typically cause a slow decline in these cognitive functions; however, the progression is variable (APA, 2013).

Vascular Dementia

According to the Alzheimer's Association (2021b), vascular dementia (VaD) is the second most common type of dementia. VaD is associated with heart disease or stroke, which impair the flow of blood to the brain. These interruptions in blood flow (for example, blood clots or hemorrhages) may cause multiple strokes that cause deterioration of the brain and its functions over time. The person may experience signs of a stroke and, after some time, may regain some of that impaired function only to then have signs of another stroke, possibly with different signs and accompanying problems. Besides symptoms of dementia (impaired judgment, thought processes, and language function, as well as memory loss), the person may display other signs of vascular disease. These may include paralysis or weakness of the limbs, disorientation, movement disorders, and speech disorders, such as apraxia of speech and dysarthria (previously discussed in chapter 2).

Parkinson's Disease Dementia

Not every person diagnosed with Parkinson's disease will have dementia, but some do. The Alzheimer's Association (2021a) states that approximately 50% to 80% of persons with PD will eventually develop dementia. If they do, it will typically show up years after the physical symptoms associated with Parkinson's disease (such as tremors at rest; bradykinesia, or slow movement; and muscle rigidity) and the diagnosis of PD has been determined. Symptoms of Parkinson's disease dementia include problems with memory, concentration, and judgment; visual hallucinations; paranoid delusions; depression; agitation; and anxiety.

Frontotemporal Dementia

Frontotemporal dementia (FTD) is a group of disorders that develop because of the death of brain cells in the frontal or temporal lobes (for more information on the lobes of the brain, see chapter 5 and appendix D). These disorders do not have the prominent issues with memory that AD does. Instead, they affect language, personality, and behavior. This type of dementia is the most common type to occur in younger people, with symptoms starting between 40 and 65 years of age. Nonetheless, FTD can also develop in younger adults and those over 65.

One type of FTD is primary progressive aphasia (PPA). According to Jung, Duffy, and Josephs (2013), this dementia first causes a language disorder, such as the inability to understand what is being said or to find the words to communicate effectively. Eventually, individuals with PPA will develop loss of memory and the ability to communicate (for more information on PPA, see chapter 5).

The behavioral variant of FTD (bv-FTD) is another type. Persons with this type may show a loss of insight, significant personality changes, and disruptions in their social interactions and interpersonal skills. The initial signs may be changes in mood, motivation, and inhibition, and it may first be misdiagnosed as a psychiatric disorder, usually depression or a personality disorder. These changes gradually become noticed by relatives, coworkers, and friends as they start to adversely affect the person's work performance and personal relationships (Leyton & Hodges, 2010).

Alcohol-Related Dementia

Like *Max* in the case study at the beginning of this chapter, people who abuse alcohol may exhibit signs of dementia, usually after many years of consuming alcohol. Alcohol abuse may cause brain damage that develops because of multiple factors (for example, number of drinks per day). This type of dementia, also known as Korsakoff's syndrome, causes various behaviors that depend on the areas of the brain damaged by the abuse. Those behaviors include problems with planning and organizational skills, poor judgment and risk assessment, impulsivity, irritability and emotional outbursts, problems with attention and reasoning, socially inappropriate behavior, and insensitivity to others' feelings (Alzheimer's Association, 2021a–c).

What Are Some Physical and Social-Emotional Changes for Persons with Dementia?

Dementia is predominantly a disorder experienced by older individuals, typically defined as at least 65 years of age. According to Besdine (2019), this is the age often used to refer to older individuals; however, most people do not need special geriatric care until age 70, 75, or even 80 years or age and older. Communication breakdowns caused by typical aging make the effects of the cognitive decline seen in dementia even worse. These communication breakdowns experienced by the aged population, especially those living in nursing homes, may have several concerning side effects that affect your family member's physical and social-emotional well-being, including loss of independence, livelihood and social roles, physical attractiveness and grooming skills, energy, friends and family, and familiar environments (Santo Pietro & Ostuni, 2003).

What Are the Three Stages of Alzheimer's Disease and How Does Communication Change at Each Stage?

There are distinct stages of loss of the ability to communicate in AD. Within these early, middle, and late stages, there are marked changes in communication and social skills as the deterioration continues (Hickey & Bourgeois, 2018).

Early Stage (Mild Alzheimer's Disease)

In the early stage, your loved one may have difficulty remembering words or finding them for use during conversation. Yet, they will continue to use the rules of our language, such as correct grammar and sentence structure. They will understand abstract thoughts and concepts, such as metaphors ("It's raining cats and dogs!"). They will also be able to engage in complicated conversations. Your loved one will continue to be able to read aloud and comprehend reading, as well as perform simple writing tasks. They will continue to understand concrete language and short yes or no questions (Hickey & Bourgeois, 2018). They may lose some long-term and short-term memory, have trouble recalling recently acquired information, and have difficulty remembering a five-item list. In this stage, these impairments may not be noticeable in their conversations.

Your loved one may lose the ability to understand speech in noisy or distracting environments. They may lose the ability to take part in conversation as before and display an inability to come up with topics. They may also lose the ability to understand rapidly spoken speech or to find words as quickly as before. Your loved one may also substitute related words for the intended word (for example, door for window) but can correct these substitutions in this early stage. Socially, in this early stage, your loved one may lose the ability to stay on topic or control their argumentativeness or anger. The person's speech may appear rude, and they may be unable to pay attention to you for more than a few minutes (Santo Pietro & Ostuni, 2003).

Middle Stage (Moderate Alzheimer's Disease)

According to Hickey and Bourgeois (2018), in the middle stage, your loved one may have increasing difficulty finding the words they intend to say, exhibit breakdowns in the ability to complete what they intended to say, and speak sentences that lack information or content. The person in this stage may continue to lose even more short-term and long-term memory abilities. They will have difficulty understanding multistep commands and will not remember the information after it is told to them. The person with moderate AD will lose abstract vocabulary, concepts, or the names of people less familiar to them. They may not remember a three-item list (for example, bread, milk, and cheese) or follow three-step commands (for example, open the door, turn on the light, and walk in), and will not recall information after it is told to them.

In this middle stage, your loved one may lose the ability to understand long conversations and pay attention in the presence of noise or distraction; however, they will continue to follow short conversations on topics that pertain to them, such as hobbies or political beliefs. The person may also exhibit the inability to read facial cues (for example, understanding surprise or sadness on someone's face). They may lose the ability to find words previously in their vocabulary and the ability to self-correct. Speech will become less free flowing and may contain more pauses and sentence fragments.

Socially, in the middle stage, this person may lose the ability to see things from another's perspective and become more self-centered. They may ask fewer questions and take part less often in conversation. When the person engages in conversation, they may appear rude. They may make eye contact less and have more difficulty using the appropriate language in social situations (Hickey & Bourgeois, 2018).

Late Stage (Severe Alzheimer's Disease)

In the last stage, your loved one may lose the ability to express their needs and wants. According to Hickey and Bourgeois (2018), a person with severe AD will frequently use repetitive and disruptive utterances or be nearly mute as they enter the end stage of the disease. They will exhibit a lack of awareness and loss of the ability to understand the meanings of most words. They may also be unaware when someone is speaking to them. Socially, they will lose the desire to communicate or have social interactions.

How Does the Progression of Dementia Affect Communication?

Caregivers and close family members will soon be able to recognize distinct changes in the person's communication style as their disease process and dementia continues to progress. One of these changes is the use of the same utterance repeatedly (for example, "Look out now!"). Another is the use of "empty speech." This can happen when a person speaks in general terms because they cannot think of specific words (for example, "Give me that thing," for "Give me the remote control"). They may also use words that are similar to the words intended, or they may say the opposite of what they meant (for example, door for window).

Within their conversations, persons with dementia may also break conversational rules we observe innately by interjecting with rude or self-centered utterances. Your loved one may cry, swear, walk away, or make totally unrelated comments during a conversation. Also, fortunately, within their conversations, there may be periods, or windows, of awareness or understanding in which they suddenly remember things or can clearly engage in conversation about a topic that seemed to be long forgotten. While there is a long list of skills that persons with dementia lose the ability to perform as their disease progresses, there are also abilities and skills that remain intact until much later in the disease course.

What Are Some Preserved Communication Abilities in Persons with Dementia?

Persons with dementia have many communication skills that remain preserved. The six abilities described below are nearly always preserved, even in the later stages of the disease (Santo Pietro & Ostuni, 2003).

1. Use of procedural memories: While people with dementia begin to lose memory for words, information, and events, their memory for how to perform familiar tasks, such as locking a door and driving a car, may be preserved. This type of memory is called procedural memory. More examples of tasks associated with procedural memory include reading the newspaper, serving coffee, setting a table, playing the piano, or dancing (see chapter 8).

Unfortunately, these preserved procedural memories are also present in people who may get into a car and become lost because they cannot remember how to return home. The Silver Alert program was created in response to this issue with the elderly and with people who have dementia. Silver Alert is a public notification system implemented in thirty-seven states and the District of Columbia to broadcast information when a senior citizen, especially one with dementia, is missing. It implements alerts across numerous media outlets (for example, variable-message signs on roadways, alerts on television stations). For more information on Silver Alert; the Wanderer Reunification Program, a program that provides help in returning a loved one who has wandered away; and ways to lower the chances of your loved one wandering, see the Alzheimer's Association website and the Alzheimer's Family Organization in the list of sources at the end of this chapter.

2. The ability to access early life memories: Research has found that a person's earliest memories may be hard wired, so they may still remember these memories, even into the later stages of their disease. Several recreational activities can capitalize on these memories to create pleasant feelings and bring comfort to your loved one. Simple Pleasures is an example of one of these activities (Hickey & Bourgeois, 2018). It involves the creation of handmade items to use during interactions with nursing home residents. Using these Simple Pleasures decreases isolation and inactivity. An example provided by Hickey and Bourgeois (2018) was the creation of a memory box for a patient who had worked in an auto body shop for

many years. Inside the box were toy cars, pictures of tools, and other items that would allow him to reminisce about his days as a mechanic and provide positive, calming feelings in this person.

3. The ability to recite, read aloud, and sing with good pronunciation and grammar: Researchers studying the language of individuals with dementia have long known that their use of proper grammar remains (Santo Pietro & Ostuni, 2003). Frequently, they can still recite prayers, sing their favorite songs, read aloud a greeting card, and respond appropriately to social greetings. This remaining language ability can bring much joy and comfort to the person with dementia and their loved ones.

4. The ability to engage in social rituals: Your loved one with dementia may still use social niceties and greetings well into the middle stage of the disease. They may still engage in small talk (for example, "How's the weather?"), exchange social greetings ("good morning"), and accept compliments ("thank you"). Your loved one may also show the ability to take turns in conversation well into the middle stage.

5. The desire for interpersonal communication: Until the late stages of dementia, individuals may continue to desire communication. Losing that desire may show that your loved one is moving into a more severe stage of the disease.

6. The desire for interpersonal respect: Persons with dementia retain the desire for interpersonal respect. Signs of this are the resentful behaviors they may display if treated poorly by those in their environment. The perception of being treated with a lack of respect includes such behaviors as having caregivers who talk with them

as if they are a child, being ignored, and receiving medical treatment without explanation (Santo Pietro &
Ostuni, 2003). It is important to use the skills that your
loved one still has to communicate in the best manner.

Let's turn now to some general guidelines and specific techniques to
help make communication more effective and meaningful with your
loved one with dementia.

What Are Some General Guidelines for More Effective Communication with Persons with Dementia?

Use adult language: Use an adult communication style
to help your loved one maintain self-respect. They may
respond negatively when you address them as if they were a
child, no matter how kindly you approach them.

Maintain eye contact: Use nonverbal cues whenever possible. Maintaining eye contact is vital for communication. If
the person with dementia is not looking at you, first establish eye contact by touching their arm or calling their name
before you speak.

Use visual cues when possible: Research into the communication styles of individuals with dementia reveals that
they respond to visual communication longer than to spoken communication. Using written words presented in large
print so they are more easily seen is helpful, as reading is
frequently preserved in individuals with dementia. Gestures, pictures, and facial expressions can also assist you or
your loved one's ability to communicate more effectively.

Avoid saying, "Don't you remember?": Reminders that
your loved one with dementia is steadily losing their mem-

ory are stressful to both them and you, the caregiver. Constantly questioning them will not bring the memories back.

Do not shout: If the loved one does not have a hearing deficit, a loud tone of voice may frighten them or make them defensive. Persons who have a hearing impairment also may have tinnitus (ringing in the ears) or recruitment (impaired perception of soft noises, while they perceive loud noises at their actual level of loudness). Because either of these conditions may worsen when there is shouting, to shout may cause your loved one extreme stress.

Do not interrupt: Avoid interrupting unless absolutely necessary. Interrupting the individual, either during an attempt to communicate or while performing a task, may cause them to forget what they wanted to say or what they were doing.

Avoid competition: Avoid the competing signals of a television or other conversations when attempting to talk with the person. Speak to them face to face in a quiet environment.

Use a calm, reassuring tone of voice: Your voice should reflect a pleasant tone, so the person will want to listen to what you are saying. People with dementia respond to emotional tone, so communicate in a reassuring and comforting tone, not an angry or agitated one.

Do not talk about the person in their presence: Even those in the last stage of dementia may have windows of lucidity. To speak negatively or sarcastically about them to others while in their presence may influence the person to react negatively.

Allow extra time for the person to respond: Your loved one may understand and process information more slowly. If given enough time, they may surprise you with an appropriate response.

Keep your explanations short: The person may be able to complete tasks if you break them down into short steps (for example, "Pick up your fork, please"; "Try the mashed potatoes").

Be realistic in your expectations: Be patient with your loved one's honest efforts to communicate. You should address their strengths.

Realize that catastrophic reactions and crying out might not be manipulative: Catastrophic reactions, such as shouting and crying out, are not attempts to manipulate. These are most likely the person's inability to communicate needs, the expression of frustration at not being able to communicate these needs, or an episode of feeling overwhelmed.

Be willing to talk about old times: Allow your loved one to reminisce about their early years. Giving them time to share these memories may help them perform better in the present.

Listen carefully to what may appear to be rambling by your loved one: Many times, persons with dementia may appear to have utterances they repeat consistently and that appear meaningless. When you pay attention to this rambling, however, you may discover a theme and meaning in what they are saying and be able to respond accordingly and with reassurance to your loved one.

Use touch: You can communicate affection, humor, support, and reassurance through touch, even into the last stage of dementia.

Pay attention to nonverbal communication: Frequently, persons with dementia can still express themselves through nonverbal communication. Pay attention to their gestures, smiles, nods, and frowns.

Use simple words and short sentences: Your loved one with dementia will better understand simpler and shorter messages (Santo Pietro & Ostuni, 2003).

What Are Some Specific Conversation Techniques for Persons with Dementia?

People can use these techniques in their everyday interactions with persons with dementia (Santo Pietro & Ostuni, 2003):

A choice question: Giving the person a choice between two acceptable alternatives may enhance their ability to make choices, whether it be objects, activities, words, or opinions. Persons with dementia may respond better to questions given a choice of two answers instead of trying to come up with the answer on their own. An example might be "Charlotte, do you want to wear your red shoes or your white shoes?" as opposed to "Charlotte, what color shoes do you want to wear with this dress?" Persons with dementia may be unable to give the elaborate answers that open-ended questions require, so they may say nothing. This technique of giving choices can also be effective in avoiding a confrontation and managing a person's behavior. Instead of saying, "Roger, put on your jacket," one could say "Roger, would you like help putting on your jacket, or can you put it on yourself?" When a person feels they have some control over what is happening, they are less likely to resist or become combative.

Matching comment or association: Persons with dementia frequently will make a comment and then not follow up with another response to continue the conversation. One likely reason for this is they may have already forgotten the comment. A technique for maintaining the conversation is to reply with a matching comment or an association, rather than a follow-up question. An example of a response to the comment "I like mashed potatoes" could be "You like mashed potatoes? I do, too. I also like french-fried potatoes." This might give them the opportunity to respond with "I like hamburgers." Then you could continue the conversation with these and other associated topics.

Closure: Closure is a technique in which the speaker provides all but the last one to two words in a sentence, and the person fills in the blanks. Most persons will respond to this cue, and even those in the later stage of the disease may respond if the topic is familiar enough. An example could be "Please help me here! Your daughter's name is ——." Giving the person an introduction to the sentence will allow them time to tune in and attend to what you are saying before you present the statement requiring the missing information. This technique is helpful for practicing the vocabulary they have remaining. An example: While holding up their shirt, say "Here is your ——." We know that words practiced frequently are more likely to remain longer in a person's vocabulary as the dementia progresses.

Repair: A repair is a word or a statement that fills in some of your loved one's information or corrects some misinformation they said. For example, when a person says, "It's snowing outside," instead of your response being "No, that's not snow. It's rain. See? It's rain," try saying, "That rain is really coming down! I got all wet this morning." This way you are responding to their conversation initiation while correcting misinformation in a pleasant, nonconfrontational manner. The person could interpret the first example as a put-down and feel agitated. Repair is also an opportunity to help your loved one possibly provide more information in their empty speech. An example: When he or she says, "It's over there," your response could be "Yes, your coffee is on the table. May I get it for you?" This way you are providing more information and viable alternatives to vague references to objects or information.

What Are the Important Take-Home Points in This Chapter?

- Dementia is a progressive disorder that can affect short-term memory, long-term memory, abstract thinking, judgment, and language.

- There are different types of dementia (for example, Alzheimer's, frontotemporal, alcohol-related). The dementia associated with AD is the most common.

- Your loved one most likely wants and needs to communicate, despite experiencing progressively deteriorating communication skills.

- You can enhance your conversations with your loved one by focusing on abilities preserved until the late stages of the disorder, such as referring to their early life memories; engaging in social rituals, such as "How are you today?"; and asking them to read aloud or sing.

- There are guidelines to enhance your ability to communicate with your loved one, such as not shouting, not interrupting, allowing more time for a response, and being realistic in your expectations of their response to you.

- Your loved one may still be able to enjoy these happy and interactive moments of their life. Your ability to appreci-

TABLE 6.1. *Specific Conversation Techniques for Persons with Dementia*

TECHNIQUE	DESCRIPTION	PURPOSE	EXAMPLE
Choice question	Offer a choice between two acceptable alternatives	To avoid possible confrontation	"Would you like apple pie or pumpkin pie?"
Matching comment or association	Respond to the person's comment with a matching comment or association	To maintain the conversation when the person makes a comment and then appears to have forgotten	Match the person's comment "I like pumpkin pie" with "You like pumpkin pie? I like pumpkin pie, too."
Closure	After an introductory sentence, provide all but the last few words of the next sentence	To allow the person to practice remaining vocabulary	"I know you like pie. I believe your favorite pie is _____."
Repair	Provide a word or statement that fills in some of the person's vague information or corrects misinformation	To provide more information and possible alternatives	When they say, "I like that," the response would be "Yes, I know you like pumpkin pie. Would you like some pumpkin pie?"

ate those moments with them will enhance communication with your loved one and create periods of powerful connection and great enjoyment between you.

In conclusion, being bogged down with feelings of sadness and negativity when dealing with your loved one with dementia can cause you to have difficulty communicating with them. Persons with dementia can still enjoy happy moments of their lives. They can still enjoy many of the same social activities as before, especially in the early stage, such as attending family dinners, church activities, or going to weekly bingo games. In the later stages, you may incorporate activities that help them reminisce about the past, such as looking at family albums or pictures of days gone by. You might assist them by creating a memory book that contains the names and pictures of family members and important people they interact with daily (Bourgeois, 2014). You might also consider placing large labels on items used regularly (for example, signs for "Bathroom" on the bathroom door or "Fridge" on the refrigerator) and reinforce naming these items each time they use them.

While participating in some of the activities suggested above, it is also important that caregivers of persons with dementia continue to practice self-care. Take time for yourself, continue the activities that enhance your own life, and reach out for help when needed. Taking care of yourself will improve your ability to enjoy the periods of better understanding and responding to your loved one who has dementia. You will find more information on caring for yourself, the caregiver, in chapter 7.

REFERENCES

Alzheimer's Association. (2021a). *Parkinson's disease dementia*. Retrieved February 4, 2021. https://www.alz.org/alzheimers-dementia/what-is-dementia /types-of-dementia/parkinson-s-disease-dementia.

Alzheimer's Association. (2021b). *Vascular dementia*. Retrieved February 4, 2021. https://www.alz.org/alzheimers-dementia/what-is-dementia/types -of-dementia/vascular-dementia.

Alzheimer's Association. (2021c). *What is Alzheimer's disease?* Retrieved February 4, 2021. https://www.alz.org/alzheimers-dementia/what-is -alzheimers.

American Psychiatric Association (APA) (2013). *Diagnostic and statistical manual of mental disorders* (5th ed.). APA.

Besdine, R. W. (2019, April). *Introduction to geriatrics*. Merck Manual Professional Version. https://www.merckmanuals.com/professional/geriatrics /approach-to-the-geriatric-patient/introduction-to-geriatrics.

Bourgeois, M. (2014). *Memory and communication aids for people with dementia*. Health Professions Press.

Hickey, E. M., & Bourgeois, M. S. (Eds.) (2018). *Dementia: Person-centered assessment and intervention* (2nd ed.). Taylor and Francis.

Jung, Y., Duffy, J. R., & Josephs, K. A. (2013). Primary progressive aphasia and apraxia of speech. *Seminars in Neurology, 33*(4), 342–47. https://doi .org/10.1055/s-0033-1359317.

Leyton, C. E., & Hodges, J. R. (2010). Frontotemporal dementias: Recent advances and current controversies. *Annals of Indian Academy of Neurology, 13*(6), 74–80. https://doi.org/10.4103/0972-2327.74249.

Petrac, D. C., Bedwell, J. S., Renk, K., Orem, D. M., & Sims, V. (2009). Differential relationship of recent self-reported stress and acute anxiety with divided attention performance. *Stress, 12*(4), 313–19.

Santo Pietro, M. J., & Ostuni, E. (2003). *Successful communication with persons with Alzheimer's disease: An in-service* (2nd ed.). Butterworth-Heinemann.

RESOURCES

Alzheimer's Association: https://www.alz.org

Alzheimer's Family Organization: https://alzheimersfamily.org

Alzheimer's Society: https://www.alzheimers.org.uk

Emedicine Health: https://www.emedicinehealth.com

    Dementia, Symptoms, Warning Signs, Types, Causes, and Treatment: https:// www.emedicinehealth.com/dementia_overview/article_em.htm

Johns Hopkins Medicine: https://www.hopkinsmedicine.org
  Dementia: https://www.hopkinsmedicine.org/neurology_neurosurgery
  /centers_clinics/memory_disorders/conditions/dementia.html
Mayo Clinic: https://www.mayoclinic.org
  Dementia: https://www.mayoclinic.org/diseases-conditions/dementia
  /symptoms-causes/syc-20352013
Medline Plus: https://medlineplus.gov
  Dementia: https://medlineplus.gov/dementia.html
National Institute on Aging: https://www.nia.nih.gov
  What Is Dementia? Symptoms, Types, and Diagnosis: https://www.nia.nih.gov
  /health/what-dementia
Silver Alert, Wikipedia: https://en.wikipedia.org/wiki/Silver_Alert
WebMD: https://www.webmd.com
  Types of Dementia: https://www.webmd.com/alzheimers/guide/alzheimers
  -dementia

ABOUT THE AUTHOR
Dr. Elizabeth Roberts is an Associate Professor in the Department of Speech-Language Pathology at Nova Southeastern University in Fort Lauderdale, Florida, and a corporate Speech-Language Pathologist. Her areas of focus in the university setting are adult neurogenic communication disorders, including dementia, apraxia of speech, aphasia, and traumatic brain injury. As a private practitioner, she provides training in accent modification, communication strategies for families and caregiver of persons with dementia, and business communication, as well as treatment of orofacial myofunctional disorders.

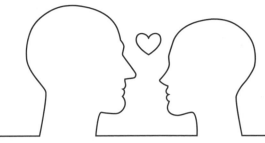

Coping and Caring for
Your Loved One and Yourself

Lea Kaploun, PhD, CCC-SLP

*Gail sat down heavily at the kitchen table with a deep sigh, numbed by
the swirling thoughts that she couldn't capture long enough to process. She
pulled out a piece of paper, really the back of an envelope, to make a list
of all the errands she needed to take care of, the bills she had to pay, and
the doctors' visits to schedule. Allowing her mind to wander for a moment,
Gail thought back to the years before Steven's stroke, when he took care of
most of those tasks. Back then, she had the time and headspace to shop for
and cook delicious, nutritious meals. She smiled to herself as she thought
about how much better her food had tasted with salt. Steven's eloquent
compliments for her savory vegetable soup had been frequent. Now, her
stress level rose when she thought about food shopping, preparation, and
cleanup. Where would she find the time? As for Steven's compliments now,
she was grateful to hear the words "thank you" from him. Aphasia and
apraxia of speech made each word he produced a treasure.*

*"Time to take my heart medication," she thought, as she remembered
her brief stay in the hospital several months before. Gail sighed again, this
time with relief as she thought of the kind medical staff that had taken
care of her. They had allowed her husband to sleep in the hospital bed*

next to hers during that stay, so she could continue to care for him while she received inpatient care for her heart condition. She couldn't imagine what he would have done if she had left him home alone. Steven could say only a few words since his stroke, and he couldn't understand many things people said, even in his first language, Russian. He couldn't prepare food for himself or even call 911 with certainty. How would he have managed? She shuddered and forced the thoughts out of her mind.

The phone rang, and Gail reached for it, thinking the caller was her daughter up north. It was the internist's office, confirming Steven's appointment for tomorrow. Gail finished the call and added another item to her "to do" list. She would need to schedule transportation from a car service to Steven's appointment. Ever since her fender bender last month, Gail had gotten behind the wheel only with reluctance and fear. She had never been much of a driver before Steven's stroke; he had always taken the wheel. Now that they were living in south Florida, a move they had made only a few months before his stroke, her lack of familiarity with the area added to her anxiety about driving. Gail admitted that she was terrified of another accident. Her heart started pounding as she thought of her growing list of things to do. Gail stopped and took some deep breaths. She knew that she needed to take care of herself so she could take care of her husband. Gail also knew she needed more help, but she didn't know where to turn.

Jack looked around the bedroom of the assisted living facility where he and Joanne had had been living for the last couple of months. What a change in their lives! Now, Joanne spent her days in a recreational room with supervision, while Jack had more time to do as he pleased. He wasn't even sure how to spend the time, but the weight of worrying about Joanne during the day was a little lighter. He felt relieved of some of the boulder he had been carrying. Jack and Joanne still shared a bedroom at the facility at night. He wasn't sure that was the best arrangement. He worried that she'd fall if she got out of bed during the night, which she sometimes did.

Mealtimes were still challenging, even without Jack having to cook or shop for food. When Jack sat with Joanne for dinner, he found the meal stressful. Joanne couldn't remember what to do with the cutlery, and she would sometimes use her hands to eat, making a mess at which the old Joanne would have cringed.

Jack thought back to when Joanne first had a stroke. At that time, she had struggled with speaking because of aphasia, but otherwise she had managed well at home. It had taken him a while to realize that Joanne was slowly getting worse instead of improving. Over the years, she had shown increasing difficulty following her routine, preferring to sit on the couch and watch TV. She continued to get speech therapy, but she was talking less, getting more confused, and taking part less in her favorite activities. She would get frustrated when Jack did not understand what she wanted, but she did not seem to make strong efforts to clarify. When he asked her where she wanted to go for dinner, Joanne wouldn't respond with an option. When he offered choices, she would indicate one choice when she meant the other. When he asked her yes or no questions to help her choose, she'd confuse the words yes and no in her response. Jack had gotten increasingly frustrated with their communication breakdowns. It was not until an incident in the bathroom, however, that he finally recognized that Joanne's problem went well beyond difficulty communicating. He had watched her stand in front of the bathroom sink, staring at her toothbrush, clearly confused about what to do with it. That was the first time he had used the term dementia.

Lately, he used the word dementia more often. He was getting used to the idea that his wife struggled with many aspects of her life, though he seemed to find it more frustrating than she did. When he got used to her decreased level of function, her skills deteriorated further. Jack was grateful for what Joanne could still enjoy, but he grappled with guilt as he sought to spend more time away from her.

———

What Are Some Ways That Coping May Be Difficult for a Caregiver?

If you are reading this chapter, you are likely either living with, related to, or taking part in the care of someone with a communication disorder. You might relate to some aspects of one or both of those stories. While their names have been changed to protect their privacy, the couples and their stories are real. Both *Jack* and *Gail* faced difficult situations that they did not expect. *Gail* had looked forward to retirement with *Steven*, unprepared to take on responsibilities he had shouldered in their marriage. Isolation exacerbated *Gail's* caregiver burden because of the physical distance from family support. *Jack* had more resources to turn to for support, but dealing with the changes in his wife still felt painful and aggravating.

Your experience might differ in many ways from each of these couples. The nature and type of your relationship might not be similar. In fact, you might not even be related to the person with difficulty communicating. In choosing to read this chapter, however, you have likely experienced some frustration in communication. Your role in relation to the person with the communication challenge might have changed, leaving you feeling frustrated. You might have experienced some strong emotions that were hard to handle as you tried to cope with the change in your life and that of your loved one.

My goal in this chapter is to share some ideas for smoothing the path to coping with this change in your life. While I write this chapter from the perspective of a health care professional who has been treating and counseling adults with communication disorders for many years, including *Steven* and *Joanne* and their families, I can also relate to the experience personally. I watched my father struggle with Parkinson's disease for years and experienced the impact it had on him and our family. While his language skills remained intact, his increasing difficulty speaking clearly and loudly enough for people to understand him proved to be challenging for him and for the rest of our family. His worsening difficulty with managing solid foods and thin liquids also required support of caregivers in providing adequate nutrition and hydration through means he could manage.

The change in your loved one may have occurred suddenly, such as from a stroke or other acquired brain injury, or gradually, such as from a degenerative disease like Parkinson's or Alzheimer's disease. In either case, that change may affect not only communication skills, but movement, meal management, and other aspects of life. These may include loss of livelihood; isolation from friends or from the world at large during periods of viral outbreak, as Covid-19 presented; a diminished role within the family and community; physical dependence for managing self-care; and many other areas. The feeling of sadness you are likely to experience is a normal and appropriate part of the grieving process, as you recognize your loved one's deficits and adjust to them. Sadness is one of the many emotions you may currently feel or will feel as you process this loss with your loved one. The problems in your loved one's communication skills and other affected abilities may improve, they may be permanent, or they may worsen. Your experience of grief as you try to cope with any of those possibilities is reasonable.

Coping, whether in a productive or an unproductive way, is an attempt to reduce the level of distress a person feels in response to a difficult event or situation. The process of coping with a change in communication skills or other loss does not follow the same path for everyone. There are different stages that individuals may experience as they come to terms with shifts in various aspects of their lives. Many authors have organized these stages of coping in multiple ways, by the emotions people face and their level of acceptance of the situation. Kübler-Ross's (1969) model of the five stages of grief originally described the experience of people with terminal diagnoses. It has been adapted to reflect the experience of those who are grieving loss of other types. The stages she described include denial, anger, bargaining, depression, and acceptance. Denial involves perceiving reality differently from its true form, when reality is too painful to face. As denial fades, anger may arise. A higher power, people, or the situation may become the target of that anger. Bargaining, the next stage, involves hope that some negotiation, such as improving your behavior, might help avoid the cause of grief. Depression may follow, and it can present as hopelessness, apathy, or even possibly suicidal thoughts. At the stage of acceptance, a person comes to terms with reality. You can read more about these stages at Grief.com (https:// grief.com/the-five-stages-of-grief/). Matson and Brooks (1977), in their work with people living with multiple sclerosis, described the process that a person may experience in developing the confidence to deal with the difficult situation at hand. Their stages of coping include denial, resistance, affirmation, and integration. The journey may begin with difficulty acknowledging the problem. Resistance involves a plan to defeat the problem. Affirmation entails acknowl-edging but feeling consumed by the problem. At the stage of integra-tion, a person begins to put the challenging situation in perspective. Whether you find that your experience matches aspects of these mod-els or takes a different path, you can likely relate to some emotions associated with the journey of coping with disorder.

Keep in mind that the process may not follow the same path for everyone. People can face earlier stages of coping even after having processed their loss at some level. As people get more comfortable with a situation, they may feel more equipped to handle issues that arise and may not need to hide from them. Even after moving on from denial to more accepting stages of coping, a negative change in the situation may trigger new feelings of fear, pain, or grief. The people who had already experienced later stages of coping may find them-selves back in an earlier stage, coping again with the new changes.

For example, if a loved one was using a cane but now needs a walker, this change can trigger a new cycle of coping for everyone involved. When people with worsening Parkinson's disease find that their strategies for improving speech clarity no longer work because the disease is progressing, feelings of anger and frustration can arise as they did when their speech first became less clear. Sometimes, it's not even a new negative change that triggers the need for coping again. It might be another milestone that the family hasn't yet faced after the onset of the disorder. Holidays during the first year after onset of the communication impairment can be especially hard. Memories of interaction and traditions on those holidays from before onset can be painful in contrast to the current situation. People might think they have finished coping with the changes involving holidays after their first Thanksgiving with their loved one with aphasia. When New Year's comes around, however, they find themselves reeling from grief again.

Each stage of deterioration in *Joanne's* communication skills triggered a flood of emotion and a return to earlier stages of coping for *Jack*, as he again processed his feelings and recognized the changes taking place. When *Jack* got used to *Joanne's* method of communication, her level of understanding, and the amount of support she needed to get her needs met, her skill level deteriorated, and he again questioned why she struggled to understand him. While his process quickened with subsequent changes, *Jack* still needed to repeat the stages of coping with each new level of deterioration.

Research and the personal experiences of many individuals support the strategies for coping in this chapter. That doesn't mean that all the strategies will work for you. Try a strategy or two and see if they help. I hope you'll find at least one idea that can support your coping process with the changes that are taking place or have taken place in your life.

How Can You Acknowledge Your Emotions?

Believe it or not, unlike your teeth, which will eventually go away if you don't take care of them, negative emotions don't disappear if you do not address them. They fester and present in different ways. Those negative emotions may show in a burst of anger at the dry cleaner who is taking too long to find your suit, tears that flow unexpectedly during a casual conversation with a friend, or an empty half-gallon container of ice cream that you bought yesterday, among other surprising presentations.

People facing loss show or report feeling grief, anger, guilt, confusion, and inadequacy, among other negative emotions (Luterman, 2017). Recognizing those emotions is the first step in processing them, so that you don't act on them without being aware. Processing negative emotions as part of coping doesn't make them disappear. They just become more manageable, to make room for more positive emotions.

Family members experience many common emotions in dealing with the onset of a communication disorder. People report grief from the profound loss that results from the disorder. They might mourn the loss of their envisioned and planned future or losing the way they related to each other. A couple might have been saving up for years for retirement with a plan to travel the world, only to find that the person with communication impairment and other deficits needs those funds for treatment and home care, in addition to possibly having limited mobility for travel. Another couple might have looked forward to making up for all the time spent apart when working long days and focusing on parental responsibilities, only to find that in their empty nest, communication with each other is more frustrating than satisfying. They might have planned on evenings spent at favorite restaurants, only to find that difficulty managing meals and swallowing changes those plans. A couple might have been comfortable with specific roles within the household, extended family, and their own relationship. The change in communication, besides other changes, may require stepping away from a level of comfort to develop new roles and interaction styles.

Often, people living with someone with a communication disorder feel angry, whether about the situation, at the person with the communication disorder, or at themselves. They feel angry about real or perceived wrongs committed in dealing with the issues at hand. The caregivers might resent their loved one for abandoning them to deal with responsibilities alone. Frustration with the delays caused by communication breakdowns and with every other task affected by the disability takes a toll on the caregivers, and patience can wear thin. Some people feel guilty about not doing enough for the person with the disorder. They might feel guilty about getting angry when they feel overburdened. Some caregivers direct their anger inward when they regret behaving impatiently or angrily with the person with the communication impairment.

Inadequacy is another powerful emotion for people coping with the unfamiliar territory of communication impairment and its consequences. People might wish that a hero could rescue them from the situation, that someone could wave a wand and make it all go away. Vulnerability in facing the unknown with inadequate information, confusion about conflicting information or about decision making, and many other emotions could arise in coping with the onset of a communication impairment (Luterman, 2017).

Some people are uncomfortable thinking about and facing their emotions, let alone talking about them. Some feel it doesn't do any good to talk about situations that can't change. If you feel that way, you might consider that talking about your intense emotions sometimes makes them more manageable. An emotion might become more intense or fester when it's kept inside. Speaking about it can release some of its intensity, making the emotion take on more realistic proportions. Sharing your emotion with another person can also release some of the shame it can cause (Brown, 2010). Sharing might help you develop insight about why you feel that way, even if the person you talk to cannot give you any advice about how to manage your emotions. If you work through your emotions with someone who can provide some insight into dealing with them, you might ease your burden even more.

I'm not suggesting that you must speak to a mental health professional, though I recommend it if you feel that you could benefit from professional support. Mental health professionals, whether psychologists or other types of counselors, receive training to support you with as little interference as possible from their own issues. They can help you develop insight about your personal journey and can provide tools and strategies for coping with painful experiences. Social workers support people with information and resources in the community and provide a sounding board to process feelings, so that people can function better in their social role and environment. If talking to a mental health professional doesn't feel comfortable to you, consider talking to a close friend, a clergy person, or other members of a support group. You might even find that the person you confide in also wants to share some emotions, and you can provide support to each other. Being on the giving end, too, can make receiving help a little easier.

If access to emotional support is limited by your physical isolation, whether because of your concern regarding leaving your loved one alone or because access to mental health professionals presents a greater challenge during times of medical isolation, there are alternatives available. For your concern regarding leaving your loved one home alone, you might ask a friend to come visit for a couple of hours while you step out. During times of social isolation when in-person visits are limited, you might consider a telehealth visit to a mental health professional via computer or phone.

Emma, one of the participants in our caregiver support group, shared that she felt like punching a wall sometimes, in frustration with the communication breakdowns with her husband, who has aphasia. She reported feeling resistance to speaking to a psychologist, acknowledging her perception of stigma attached to that idea. She recognized, however, that she was not getting enough insight from attending the group support sessions. She finally reported back to the group that she had attended a couple of sessions with a therapist, and it "wasn't so bad!" Emma noted her positive experience having someone truly hear what she was experiencing and offer some helpful strategies for coping with her frustration.

How Can You Focus on the Positive, Including Your Own Strengths?

Every situation has positive and negative aspects. Sometimes, people focus on the negative aspects to the degree that they no longer see the positive. Taking the time to look for the positive in a situation doesn't mean that the negative no longer exists; it just takes a back seat for a little while. Believe it or not, focusing on the positive regularly can help you train your brain to do so, which can relieve anxiety and help you make clearer decisions (Wehrenberg, 2008). If your loved one had a stroke and now has aphasia, focusing on their level of communication skills compared to their prestroke ability is likely to leave you weighed down by their level of loss. Instead, think about your loved one's level of impairment right after the stroke and compare that with their current ability. Look at how far they have progressed and call attention to their and your contribution to the progress that has taken place (Holland & Nelson, 2014). You aren't fooling yourself by focusing on the positive changes that have taken place. Instead, you are choosing to devote more mental and emotional energy to thoughts and feelings that are realistic and hopeful.

Take the time to think about daily gifts in your life. Gifts might not only be abilities or objects. They can be the people around you. Who has stepped up to help in ways you would not have expected? Which of your loved one's spared skills makes functioning easier? What are you thankful for in your current situation? Consider making a daily list of things in your life for which you are grateful. Avoiding repetition of previously listed items can encourage you to broaden the range of your ideas. Think about the world around you and the world inside you. For the world around you, options can be as detail focused as the beautiful shade of red of the changing leaves on the maple tree outside your kitchen window, or as general as the wondrous universe. For your inner world, you might focus on your sense of smell and its contribution to your enjoyment of the bittersweet scent of freshly brewed coffee or more broadly recognize the enormity of the gift of life. You might consider expressing gratitude in a specific manner to a person who helps you, such as thanking the aide who consistently comes on time for their shift, noting how their dependability eases your mind. The more attention you give to the process and the more detail you add to your appreciation, the stronger your feelings of gratitude can grow. When *Gail*, the woman from the first story, became anxious about her situation and could focus only on its negative aspects, we talked about using this exercise. She began creating a daily list of items for which she was grateful and reported that her level of optimism increased.

Finally, look at your own strengths. What do you bring to the situation that helps you manage better? Which of your gifts contributes to your loved one's ability to thrive? People often have an easier time pointing out their flaws than recognizing their strengths. Martin Seligman, a well-known clinician and author on the topic of positive psychology, worked with Christopher Peterson to develop an assessment tool to help people determine their relative strengths from among twenty-four character traits that people show. The assessment, called the VIA Survey of Character Strengths, takes a bit of time to complete (there are 240 questions!), but the results show five top strengths for the test taker. Focusing on stronger character traits can help a person use those strengths more in their inner and interpersonal life. When a person recognizes and uses those strengths, they feel better about themselves and their situation. For example, if curiosity is one of your strengths, think about how you feel when you use your curiosity to learn more about people and ideas. If compassion, loving, or seeking justice is one of your best assets, how can you use that character trait to live your life more fully? Recognize how you feel when you use that strength and take time to exercise it more in your daily life with your loved one. You might find the experience invigorating. (If you are interested in taking the VIA Survey of Character Strengths, you can find it at the University of Pennsylvania's Authentic Happiness website, https://www.authentichappiness.sas .upenn.edu/, under the link for "Questionnaires.") You might even consider giving the survey in a modified form to your loved one with aphasia, dementia, or other acquired brain injury or degenerative disease. Try showing them individual cards indicating each strength for them to choose from or even having a conversation about each strength, to the degree that your loved one can understand. This can help them recognize their own strengths and try to tap into them. When the person with a communication impairment taps into their strengths, they can reap the benefits of positivity, too.

When *Jack*, the caregiver from our second story, completed a modified form of the VIA survey, he recognized that one of his strengths is loyalty. He noted that *Joanne* had taken care of him for many years of their marriage, and now it was his turn to take care of her. When he talked about how important it was for him to show loyalty to *Joanne*, he sat up straighter in his chair, showing a renewed sense of purpose in fulfilling his role in their daily life.

How Can You Keep Your Expectations Realistic?

When catastrophe strikes, people sometimes have difficulty facing reality. They might react in different ways that reflect the struggle to see the situation with inner calm. Some people become highly emotional, making it difficult for them to see the full picture with any hope for the future. They may focus on worst-case scenarios and panic, instead of problem solving to address the issues that arise. Other people turn off emotion completely and get caught up in information like diagnoses, prognosis, and treatment options. Don't get me wrong—there's nothing wrong with wanting and needing that information. Sometimes, however, people use the pursuit of that information as an escape or distraction from facing their emotions. They may perceive their emotions as too frightening to face, but hiding from their emotions doesn't allow them to process and address the full situation with all its subtleties.

Developing healthy ways of coping with and accepting the disorder involves allowing yourself to feel negative feelings as well as processing the information presented, in order to maintain realistic expectations about your loved one, yourself, and the situation. Some strategies to help you develop and maintain realistic expectations include the following:

> **Educate yourself about your loved one's disorder.** This
> may help you predict areas of possible struggle in over-
> all function and communication. Ask the medical doctor
> and rehabilitation professionals about what is appropriate
> to expect in movement, sleep patterns, pain, speech-lan-

guage, swallow skills, and other changes seen with the onset or progression of a disorder. This educational process does not take place in a single session. You might take in some information during one interaction with a health care professional and then need some information repeated, or you might encounter issues after your initial consultation. Take notes when you get information, ask for written handouts to read later, and don't be afraid to ask the professional to clarify if you don't understand what you're told. When you catch yourself getting frustrated that your loved one is not meeting your expectations, review the information from the professionals to check yourself. For example, consider viewing a website that shows some simulation examples of communication breakdowns that take place with aphasia (for example, see the "Aphasia Simulations" at http://www.vohaphasia.org/simulation/). The simulations can help you take the perspective of your loved one with communication deficits and can also help you recognize that your loved one's errors are consistent with the diagnosed communication disorder. You might even consider practicing some exercises to simulate a language disorder yourself, to imagine how you would want others to respond to you.

The health care professional will hopefully share some strategies with you to support your loved one's function and communication. For example, if your husband with aphasia struggles with answering yes or no questions and gives an answer different from his intended response, your speech-language pathologist can show you some alternative ways of asking questions. If your loved one's voice is sometimes too soft for you to hear, an amplification device, like a portable microphone, might be handy to have around for those times. Hopefully, those strategies will help you and your loved one feel less frustrated by conversation, and your expectation of their performance will be more consistent with their ability.

Allow yourself to mourn your loved one's lost abilities. This can help you face the existing losses with more acceptance. If you recognize that you might experience wishful thinking when you want your wife to eat independently and at a steady pace, as she used to, you may need to remind yourself that this is all part of the picture of the disability and not in your control. Remind yourself that she is the same wife she was before her stroke or the progression of her physical weakness or cognitive impairment, but that the difficulties she has are part of her new normal existence. Try as you might, you can't wish that away.

Schedule less to accomplish in specified periods. Sometimes, people try to fit too much into a day, and then they get frustrated when the person with a disability can't perform to expected levels of participation. Sometimes, the expectation is not even of your loved one with a disability, but of yourself as a caregiver. There are only so many tasks that you can complete in a day and only so much that your loved one has the mental, physical, and emotional energy to accomplish. Give yourself and your loved one a break and create spaces in the day for delays in scheduling and transportation and for breathing. If you have a doctor's appointment at 11 a.m., don't schedule another appointment for 1:30 p.m., hoping to encounter an empty waiting room at the doctor's office and traffic-free highways between appointments, with no break for lunch. You won't be at your best, and neither will your loved one. If possible, try to schedule appointments for times of the day when you have more energy, and avoid times that will leave you in rush-hour traffic on the way home. If your loved one with Parkinson's disease takes medication that allows them the most movement in the early afternoon, schedule their appointments for those times, so that they will be able to take part more fully during their appointments and move more easily to get to and from the appointment.

Tune into your own needs to make sure you are addressing them, so that you can support your loved one effectively without cutting corners in caregiving. If you have not had your regular morning coffee, if you need to take care of something for yourself, or if you are not feeling your best, consider the impact of those factors on your interaction with your loved one. While you sometimes need to take care of your family before you get to meet all your own needs, be realistic about the possibility that you might be a little more abrupt and impatient. Forgive yourself for not being as tolerant as you are with a full night's sleep and a strong cup of coffee.

Accept a less-than-perfect picture. In an ideal world, you have full-time help to meet all your own needs and the needs of your loved one. You have a house stocked with fresh food all the time; time to cook nutritious and delicious meals three times a day (hey, why not a live-in chef, while we're dreaming); an empty laundry basket; a spotless and dust-free home; children who are dressed, fed, bathed, with backpacks full of completed homework and high scores on their exams; helpful neighbors; and extended family who come to help and then leave when you need space. Reality doesn't necessarily match that fantasy, and you have just so much time and energy. Something must give. Prioritize what is most important and let go of some less vital tasks, for the sake of your sanity. The laundry can wait a little longer. No one is coming over with white gloves to make sure that you have recently dusted the furniture. A meal of cheese pizza includes carbohydrate, protein, fat, and vegetable food groups!

Where Can You Find Help?

You don't have to do this alone! Even if your family is not close by or available to support you and your loved one, there are other ways to get help and different types of help that can ease the burden of caregiving. Take some time to reflect on which types of help will best ease your burden most quickly and are most easily accessible without too much effort.

Household Help

Getting someone to help with housekeeping, food shopping, and meal preparation can ease caregiver burden. If you're concerned about bringing a stranger into your home, note that some agencies perform thorough background checks on the people they hire to help in your home. You can speak to an agency administrator about their process of recruiting and checking the background of their employees. While the fees can add up, examining your budget to determine how much help you can afford can ease your mind about paying for a little help. Even having someone come every couple of weeks to clean the bathrooms or take care of other more strenuous tasks can make your life a little easier, allowing you to devote your energy to more important tasks.

While many people feel uncomfortable asking friends for help, you might find that some of your friends wish they knew how they could be useful to you. A clinician who has worked extensively with caregivers suggested keeping a pocket-sized notebook to jot down tasks for which an extra pair of hands would be valuable. If someone asks how they can be helpful to you, you can pull out the pad and give an authentic response, rather than brushing aside the offer because you can't think in the moment. If someone asks if you need anything, consider requesting that they pick up your groceries for you. Your local supermarket might even have a pick-up service, where your friend can drive up and get the packages of food you ordered without having to shop in the store. You'll have a few moments to take a breath, and your friend will feel good about being able to pitch in. Better yet, your local supermarket might have a delivery service for a nominal fee.

Respite Care

Everyone needs a break from caregiving at some point. Even a window of a few hours to play a round of golf or meet a friend at a local café can energize or soothe, as the need may be. Consider finding someone to keep your loved one company if they need supervision, whether through a reputable company that provides respite care for a fee, a community organization of volunteer companions in your area, or a friend with some free time who is comfortable interacting with your loved one with a communication impairment.

Emotional Support from Your Community

Whether an informal group of friends getting together to share what's going on or a more formal group of people who come together to give and get support, talking to other people who can relate to your experience can relieve emotional tension. You might find a support group through your local hospital, university clinic, or even on the internet. If you find that you can't get out of the house, whether for personal reasons or public health concerns, online groups might be a helpful substitute for a face-to-face group. Support groups also give you an opportunity to learn more about the disorder, treatment strategies, and methods of coping from people in a similar situation. The other group members benefit from being able to share their knowledge, and you benefit from learning from other people's creativity, experience, and even mistakes.

Although this is not true for everyone, many people who have attended our clinic's caregiver support group have shared that when their spouse had a stroke with new symptoms of communication impairment, their social group diminished in size dramatically. Whether because friends didn't know how to interact with the person with communication impairment, the situation frightened friends about the reality of illness and disability, or they didn't have patience to deal with a change in their routine, many people in their social circle seemed to disappear. Few peers stuck by and learned how to communicate with and include the person with aphasia, dementia, or other communication impairment in conversation.

Thus, besides dealing with an acquired brain injury or a degenerative disease and all its consequences, people with communication impairment and their loved ones often deal with the loss of many friends. On the other hand, the people they meet at a support group who "get it" because of their similar experiences often become their new support system, creating a social network of caring friends.

Transportation

Subsidized transportation services can be helpful in getting to scheduled medical appointments, therapy, and other destinations, especially if the person with the communication impairment has difficulty with mobility. The name of the service to contact for subsidized transportation for people with disabilities differs depending on where you live. Try contacting your local (city, county, or state) government office to find information about transport services. Rules may vary with location, and while this service is not perfect, transportation support can be helpful. Also, consider seeking transportation support from your community. Your local religious institution or community organization might help.

Physical Intimacy

While not everyone is comfortable talking about this topic, many more people are thinking about it, wishing someone could help. Especially as a spouse or significant other of someone with a communication impairment, the struggle with physical intimacy can be very real. For some, there are accompanying motor impairments that make physical intimacy more challenging. One woman whose husband had a stroke mentioned that she finds it frustrating to even slow dance with her husband, because he can't move the way he used to. For others, the lack of verbal communication makes the experience of physical intimacy less satisfying. Specialists in the field of sex therapy who work with people with disabilities can provide support in this area. Finding support to address this issue can provide relief and improved physical intimacy in relationships.

What Are Some Ways to Take Care of Myself?

Make time to take care of yourself! The safety instruction to put on your own air mask in an in-flight emergency before helping others allows you to provide support without passing out from oxygen deprivation. You can only help your loved ones if you meet your basic needs. Don't lose sight of your needs, and don't assume that because someone else would not have the same need, your need is unwarranted.

One participant from our caregiver support group made it his job to emphasize the importance of self-care to new members. He would cite statistics showing the higher incidence of caregivers in the family dying before their loved one with the disability, as a result of the caregiver's focus on caring for others at the expense of self-care. Make sure you schedule a medical wellness exam for yourself. Dental cleanings, daily exercise, nutritious meals, adequate sleep, and other forms of health maintenance are important not only for your self-care, but to make you a more effective caregiver.

Activities that reduce stress are another important aspect of self-care. What helps you destress? If it's iced coffee with a novel by your favorite author, be sure that you fit in some time for it without feeling like you are stealing time from responsibilities. If it's a game of golf with a couple of friends, schedule a round. Make sure your choices for self-care are healthy for you. A pizza pie and super-sized ice cream cone may be great for an occasional treat. But if you find yourself regularly making choices that you know are not good for your physical, emotional, or financial health, try to find more productive ways to enjoy yourself that you will feel good about, even after the experience is over. Some people enjoy retail therapy (shopping) as an outlet for stress. If you see the expenses adding up and regret some impulse purchases, you may need a different outlet for stress release. When your food choices are showing on the scale or in lab results, heed that message to choose differently in your self-care.

Whatever you choose as a method of relieving stress and self-care, make sure you fit in time for it regularly. The type of activity will differ for everyone, depending on factors such as time, personality, finances, respite support, and other factors. Some people recoup energy by taking time alone, while others seek company to relax. Destressing might mean staying home from one of your loved one's appointments and allowing someone else to accompany them to the doctor, or it might include securing paid or volunteer employment in an environment very different from your home situation. The key is that you enjoy the way you are spending time and that you don't find that time stressful.

Jack used to enjoy putting together jigsaw puzzles when he and *Joanne* lived at home. Their living space at the assisted living facility doesn't allow him to spread out the pieces for puzzles, but *Jack* has found a group of people willing to learn to play Rummikub instead.

Spend Quality Time with Your Loved One

Spending time with your loved one with a communication impairment, as you already know, is the same as it always was, in many respects. They are the same person who enjoyed sharing the activities you both enjoyed before the acquired injury to the brain or illness. The challenge now is to address the obstacles to enjoying those activities. You might feel frustrated that your Scrabble partner has trouble spelling words because of aphasia or dementia. Your bowling champion may now have weakness on one side of their body, making it hard for them to score consistent strikes as they used to. If the communication impairment or physical disability interferes with participating in those activities, consider changing those activities. If you were both active bowlers, and your loved one now presents with weakness on one side of their body, are there any accommodations that could support their bowling? Contact your local bowling alley to check. If you were Scrabble champions and aphasia or dementia now gets in the way of playing successfully, is there a modified version of the game that you can enjoy together? Perhaps it's time to consider a different game that doesn't involve high-level words, or perhaps an activity that doesn't involve language at all.

If all your shared pastimes for enjoyment are not possible, it's time to brainstorm other ways that you can both enjoy spending time together. A mix of creativity and flexibility on both your parts will help you find ways to enjoy each other. One of our group members with significant difficulty communicating took up ballroom dancing, and he and his wife enjoy their new hobby tremendously. Social groups for people with aphasia or other communication impairment may offer ideas about how to spend leisure time, either with the group or on your own. Art museums and musical concerts offer access for people using wheelchairs, gardens or malls provide chauffeured carts, and a local pier presents an opportunity for an afternoon of fishing with a picnic lunch. Check out local tourist attractions that you never made time to visit before, so you can see what interests you and your loved one. Even sitting on your patio with a glass of wine or apple cider and looking through old photo albums or digital photos with shared reminiscence can feel fulfilling. Chapter 8 covers various ways to use hobbies and interests that allow caregivers to interact and communicate with loved ones with communication impairment.

Learn Strategies to Communicate Effectively

When your loved one with a communication impairment gets stuck on words while trying to tell you something important, keeps answering "yes" when they mean "no," or doesn't understand the point you are trying to make, communication feels more frustrating than encouraging. When they try to communicate with others and get frustrated when you attempt to intervene on their behalf, you may feel at a loss about the correct way to support them. When they ask you for help in finding a word, but you do not understand what they are trying to say, you may wish you had some strategies accessible to repair those communication breakdowns.

Here, again, a combination of creativity and flexibility can help you support your loved one's communication. When the person with aphasia or dementia doesn't understand what you said, repeating your message rarely helps them. Supported conversation is a method to improve communication with your loved one, and you'll find specific strategies for using supported communication in chapter 5. The focus here is on considerations regarding the emotional impact of the language impairment on you and your loved one, so that you can more easily and calmly use strategies when needed.

Ask permission: When you see your loved one struggling to find a word and you know the word they are trying to say, before you jump in with the answer, consider asking permission. "Do you want some help, or do you want to get this on your own?" Much as you might like to help when it's so easy to do so, your loved one may want some independence in finding the word or a strategy to work around finding the word. Even if your loved one wants help, they might want an idea for a strategy, such as asking them to describe an attribute of the object they're trying to name, rather than having you say the word for them.

Plan ahead: Some situations leave less room for discussion, such as communication on the phone with an unfamiliar communication partner or a stressed, rushed situation. At those times, despite the person's preference for independence, they might need more support from you. At a quiet time together, discuss scenarios that could come up and how you might need to take the lead in communicating during those times because of the circumstances. Consider creating a signal system (for example, a hand motion, a gentle touch on the arm) so that you can both quickly agree that the situation warrants your role as communicator.

Be patient: Some situations may not be stressful or rushed, but they still create a feeling of frustration for you when your loved one wants to take more time to communicate than is comfortable for you. If you can, try to be in the moment; inhale slowly and then exhale slowly while you wait for the words to come out. Maintain eye contact and a calm facial expression so that you don't send nonverbal messages of annoyance while you stay quiet.

Get comfortable with imperfection: The person with difficulty communicating may need support to speak in front of strangers and friends. People who are unfamiliar and uncomfortable with communication impairment can convey verbal and nonverbal messages of frustration, dismay, or confusion. Exposure to that reaction can deter your loved one from attempting to communicate with others. The more comfortable you are with your loved one's style of communication and the more you advocate on their behalf to communicate through whichever method is most successful, the more empowered your loved one will feel in those speaking situations.

Be inclusive: Include your loved one in conversations with others. While your loved one may not be able to voice their opinion in the same way that they did before their acquired injury to the brain or illness, finding ways to help them participate will reduce their feelings of isolation and loss, especially regarding topics about which they are passionate. Consider strategies for eliciting comments or opinions, such as providing pen and paper for writing or drawing, asking questions that elicit the response your loved one can more easily produce, and arranging the seating so that they feel like part of the group.

Here are some key strategies to keep in mind to support your loved one's understanding of your words.

Slow down: Take the time to speak slowly, pausing after short sentences to allow processing time. Don't crowd too much information into a sentence. In addition, if your loved one is confused by your message, adding more words might make the information harder to process. Imagine pouring more water into a funnel that is already full. The added water will only spill over the sides, instead of leaving the narrow opening any faster. Instead, pause for silence; let the person try to process what you said, then when they are ready, repeat your message in a simpler way.

For example, "Debra and John are bringing their kids over for lunch tomorrow because they're in town for the weekend" can include too much information at once. Instead, try "Debra and John are coming over. [Pause] They're bringing the kids. [Pause] They're coming tomorrow for lunch. [Pause] They're in town for the weekend." If you started with the first message and confused your loved one, don't jump right into the breakdown of the sentences. Pause for a moment to let the previous message clear before giving the simpler version.

Contextual hints increase understanding: The verbal message may not be enough to get your point across. Use different methods to support your words. Pointing to an object that represents what you're talking about or using a gesture can help the person with aphasia understand your words.

For example, if you're in a café, try pointing to the pot of coffee or using the gesture for drinking when you ask what your loved one would like to drink. Perhaps a quick sketch or even the written word to accompany your spoken description can be helpful. For example, if your message, "I'll go get the car and meet you back here in five minutes" meets with a confused look, consider waiting a moment in silence to hear the message, then point to yourself and the door and say, "I'm going to the car," and then hold up your hand with extended fingers and say, "Back in five minutes."

Establish the topic clearly, then add details: Conveying the topic helps your loved one predict what you might say afterward, so that even if they don't understand every word you say, they might use their knowledge of the topic to fill in some gaps. Consider different ways of conveying the topic, such as through use of a key word, a photo, a drawing, or even pointing to an object or direction. For example, if you're about to tell a funny story about the grandchildren to your wife who has aphasia or dementia, pulling out a picture of them before you start your story can help her process the words of the story.

Check for understanding: Ask simple yes or no questions to see if your loved one understood your message. Make sure that the person with difficulty communicating has a way of conveying yes or no with relatively consistent accuracy before you depend on that method of response. Is their nod more accurate than their verbal response? Is a thumbs up/down more accurate than a nod or spoken response? Perhaps pointing to a yes or no symbol on a page might help get a more consistently accurate response. For example, after telling your loved one that you're interested in going to Olive Garden for dinner in an hour, you might ask, "Is Olive Garden okay with you?" and "Is six o'clock a good time?"

What Are the Important Take-Home Points in This Chapter?

- Allow yourself, as the caregiver of a loved one with communication impairment, to feel your negative emotions so that you can work through them; seek support from a mental health professional, a clergy person, or a friend, if needed.

- Find a support group to help you meet others who can relate to your experience.

- Focus on the positive in your life and in your loved one; recognize your strengths and how they contribute to making life better for both of you.

- Educate yourself about your loved one's disorder, so that you can maintain realistic expectations of their ability.

- Take time to address your own needs, whether physical, emotional, intellectual, spiritual, or any other need. Recognize your need for different types of help and allow others to support you.

- Discover ways to spend pleasurable time with your loved one, even if it means changing the way you engage in activities you used to enjoy together.

The role of the caregiver is multifaceted, and it's easy to feel pulled in many directions. You might even feel, sometimes, like taking care of yourself does not even earn a place on your "to do" list, let alone reach the top of the list. The challenges you encounter may require reaching into your deepest resources of strength, courage, selflessness, and faith. There is no single proven method for finding comfort and speeding the process of coping. Taking care of yourself, having realistic and optimistic expectations of yourself and your loved one, and asking for help when you need it can help you manage in this challenging, but meaningful, time. Adjusting to the new sense of normal can enable you to find satisfaction and fulfillment in your present life. Developing strategies to communicate more effectively and spending quality time together can help you achieve levels of closeness to your loved one that you never expected. I wish you joy and meaning as you navigate your journey.

REFERENCES

Brown, B. (2010). *The gifts of imperfection: Let go of who you think you're supposed to be and embrace who you are.* Hazelden.

Holland, A. L., & Nelson, R. L. (2014). *Counseling in communication disorders: A wellness perspective* (2nd ed.). Plural.

Kübler-Ross, E. (1969). *On death and dying.* Scribner.

Luterman, D. (2017). *Counseling persons with communication disorders and their families* (6th ed.). Pro-Ed.

Matson, R. R., & Brooks, N. A. (1977). Adjusting to multiple sclerosis: An exploratory study. *Social Science and Medicine, 11*(4), 245–50.

Wehrenberg, M. (2008). *The 10 best-ever anxiety management techniques: Understanding how your brain makes you anxious and what you can do to change it.* Norton.

RESOURCES

Alzheimer's Foundation of America: https://alzfdn.org
  Caregiving Resources: https://alzfdn.org/caregiving-resources/
American Association for Retired Persons: https://www.aarp.org
  National Agencies, Groups and Organizations for Caregivers: https://www
  .aarp.org/caregiving/local/info-2017/important-resources-for-caregivers
  .html
American Association of Sexuality Educators, Counselors and Therapists:
  https://www.aasect.org
American Heart Association: https://www.heart.org
  Caregiver Support: https://www.heart.org/en/health-topics/caregiver
  -support
Aphasia Corner: *Aphasia Simulations*: http://www.vohaphasia.org/simulation/
Grief.com: https://grief.com
  The 5 Stages of Grief: https://grief.com/the-five-stages-of-grief/
National Alliance for Caregiving: https://www.caregiving.org
National Stroke Association: https://www.stroke.org/en/help-and-support
  /for-family-caregivers
University of Pennsylvania, Authentic Happiness: https://www
  .authentichappiness.sas.upenn.edu
Well Spouse Association: https://www.wellspouse.org

ABOUT THE AUTHOR

Dr. Lea Kaploun is an Associate Professor in the Department of Speech-Language Pathology at Nova Southeastern University, Florida. She has worked with individuals with communication impairment due to acquired brain injury and degenerative disease for twenty-five years. Dr. Kaploun teaches graduate level courses in adult language disorders, motor speech disorders, and counseling for speech-language pathologists. She supervises individual treatment sessions for adult patients with communication disorders such as aphasia, and she has supervised NSU's Parkinson's support group and the caregiver support group for several years.

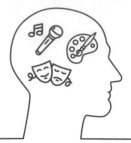

EIGHT

Using the Arts to Improve Communication and Quality of Life

Frederick DiCarlo, EdD, CCC-SLP

Imagine if someone you love or care for loses the ability to communicate. This loss is life changing, not only for the person with the communication impairment but also for the caregivers and loved ones. A communication impairment can make the person feel invisible to others. When this person has an outlet that allows expression of thoughts and feelings in other ways, however, their light and personality can shine through. This outlet allows the individual who has trouble communicating to get thoughts and feelings across to others using some form of expression. Another important result is improving their overall quality of life. Artistic expression can motivate and improve the skills of an individual with a communication impairment. The arts are a powerful tool that you can easily add to activities of daily living, weekly routines, or special occasions. Forms of artistic treatment and activities are not just for the person with a communication impairment, but also for caregivers, family, and friends who interact with the person. The arts can be a wonderful medium to reestablish bonds and shared interests between the caregivers and the person who struggles with communicating. The key element is that the caregiver, who sees the individual with the communication impairment regularly, be trained and provided with information on how to use artistic activities to improve communication. If you are reading this chapter, you are likely either living with, related to, or taking part in the care of someone with a communication impairment, who may enjoy using the arts to improve their communication and overall quality of life.

An acquired brain injury or a degenerative disease, like Parkinson's disease, may cause a person to have a communication impairment. These individuals often seek speech, language, or cognitive therapy to improve or maintain communication skills. Speech-language pathologists are finding and using creative ways to incorporate the arts, along with a person's hobbies and interests, into treatment plans. This can include activities such as singing, acting, dancing, painting, and drawing. The major goal is to make therapy fun and functional for the individual. Using the arts as a therapy tool, or as part of a home program, targets impairment areas in communication, word finding, memory, organization, and socialization. Individuals with communication impairments can become isolated, depressed, and unmotivated. Providing an outlet, using the arts specific to interests or hobbies, can help motivate the person and give them confidence in the ability to express thoughts and ideas through a chosen art form. The result is some form of communication improvement. Another important byproduct of this approach is improved quality of life for the person, family, and friends.

Artistic expression is an effective outlet for improving communication skills. Art, music, dance, and acting stimulate the entire brain, while increasing motivation and socialization. There are similarities between music therapy and speech therapy. For example, elements of music, such as melody, tempo, harmony, and rhythm, can improve expressive and receptive language skills (see chapter 5). Researchers have found that clinical treatment using musical intervention can improve speech and language skills in individuals with communication impairment (Hajjar & McCarthy, 2014). We can also expect carryover of speech and language improvement using dance, as it incorporates both music and the person's overall body movement. Art therapy can also have a positive effect with upper body movement when drawing or painting, in addition to communication. Acting improves speech by strengthening the muscles for speech and improving breath support, voice, and loudness. (We describe these topics in chapters 2 and 3.) Overall, using the arts provides results that are promising; the individual with a communication impairment is better equipped to communicate thoughts, wants, and needs for activities of daily living.

As the caregiver, you are probably looking for creative ideas that will motivate your loved one. Therefore, this chapter provides you with specific activities and strategies that incorporate the arts, including personal examples at the end of this chapter. You can include these activities and strategies in a home program, daily activities, or weekly routines, along with speech therapy or following discharge from therapy.

What Are Some Activities and Strategies That Incorporate the Arts?

Before discussing specific activities and strategies that incorporate the arts to enhance communication, there are three important ideas to cover. First are the forms of artistic expression and participation that the caregiver should understand. The forms of artistic expression and participation are *appreciation*, *re-creation*, and *creation* (Boster et al., 2018). *Appreciation* might include admiring a painting, listening to a favorite song, or clapping during a movie. Copying a painting, singing a favorite song, or reciting famous lines from a favorite movie are forms of *re-creation*. *Creation* could involve painting an original painting, writing or singing a new song, or writing a script for a play or movie. In terms of level of difficulty, appreciation requires less skill (is easier) than re-creation, which requires less skill than creation. For example, a person's skill may be such that they can only appreciate and not create. Or possibly they should re-create first before a transition to creating. Second is the level of communication impairment and the skills of the person with that impairment. These first two ideas determine how much the person will participate in the forms of artistic expression. Third is the knowledge of impairment and skills of the person, which will provide you with a guide on how to interact when using artistic activities and strategies.

The following are examples of some basic questions you should answer before engaging your loved one in an artistic activity and strategy:

- Is the person alert to the environment?

- Can the person understand what I am saying?

- Can the person follow directions and at what level?

- Can the person answer yes and no questions?

- Can the person read and understand what is being read?

- Can the person verbally or through gestures (for example, thumbs up or head nod) express themselves to convey a message?

- Can the person match a picture to a picture?

- Can the person follow a model?

- Can the person recall current or past events?

- Can the person make choices?

- Can the person use their body for writing, drawing, coloring, painting, dancing, or using a musical instrument?

- How is the person's hearing and vision?

Whatever the answers are to these questions, the caregiver needs a good understanding of the person with a communication disorder and their skill level before engaging this person in the arts. You may already have answers to some of these questions and a good overall knowledge based on being involved with your loved one and their health care rehabilitation team (for example, the speech-language pathologist, occupational therapist, or physical therapist), who may be treating your loved one or have assessed and treated them in the past. The speech-language pathologist will assist you in answering questions regarding communication, whereas the occupational therapist and physical therapist will answer questions regarding upper and lower body movement and your loved one's physical mobility for activities like dance. Consultation and collaboration with an arts-based therapist (for example, a music therapist or drama therapist) can further enhance improvement with communication, especially if the individual responds well to the arts. Another key ingredient is to determine what the person's artistic interests were in the past, before their impairment. For example, if a person loved to go to museums and admire art in the past, it is possible that they would still want to engage in that activity after their impairment. If a person never had an interest in dance in the past, however, it is unlikely they will want to dance or watch dancing after experiencing impairment.

The next portion of this chapter provides you, the caregiver, with several examples of activities and strategies to incorporate the arts into your loved one's home program, daily schedule, or routine. Please note that the examples provide you with a starting point for using the arts. You can expand on the examples to meet the needs and goals of the person with a communication impairment. All example activities can target a combination of areas of deficit in communication, word finding, memory, organization, and socialization. You should use activities that are fun, engaging, motivating, and based on the person's hobbies and interests. You can find materials for these activities in the home, local library, or online (for example, Pinterest, Google, or YouTube). Examples that follow include art, music, dance, and acting, categorized as appreciation, re-creation, and creation. As a reminder, appreciation is easiest, followed by re-creation, with creation the most difficult.

ART
Unleashing the Inner Picasso

Appreciation

Activity: Viewing paintings in a local art museum or online

Strategy: While the person is viewing each painting, ask them these types of questions:

> Is it calming?
> Is it exciting?
> What colors are in it?
> What shapes are in it?
> How does it make you feel?

Ask yourself what other questions could get the person talking.

Describe the scene of the painting. For example, what is the location? If the location is Paris, ask the person, "Have you ever visited Paris?" If the person has visited Paris, ask, "What did you think of Paris?" If the person has not visited Paris, ask "What country would you like to visit, and why?"

Alternate example: You can change the activity and strategy to include other types of paintings or sculptures that may interest the person. Also, you can modify the questions to suit the specific art form.

Your turn: Think about the person in your care and create an alternative activity and strategy that best meets the interests and needs of that person.

Re-creation

Activity: Copying line drawings or pictures of functional objects that are part of a person's daily routine (for example, dog, tennis racket, phone, purse, or wallet). Best to use a pencil for this activity; however, a fine-point marker is acceptable if preferred by the person.

Strategy: Show the person a picture you want them to name and draw. Ask the person to name the pictured object, describe it, and tell you all about it (for example, what it's used for, or where you find it). If your loved one cannot name the object in the picture, provide the first sound or first part of the word to help. Write the name of the object down if that helps. Then, ask them to draw the picture (the person should copy while the picture is in view). If the person leaves out details, point out in the picture the parts of the object missing. After the person draws the object in the picture, you can ask them to name and describe the object again.

Alternate example: You can change this activity and strategy to include a coloring activity that resembles a classic coloring book. Show the person the picture you want colored and follow the same strategies by substituting coloring for drawing.

Your turn: Think about the person in your care and create an alternative activity and strategy that best meets the interests and needs of that person.

Creation

Activity: Making an art collage

Strategy: Provide the person with a large piece of canvas art paper (16" × 20", or tape four 8" × 10" pieces of paper together), colored pencils, markers, scissors, tape, glue, and several magazines (for example, cooking magazines, grocery store flyers, *People* magazine, *Time* magazine). Ask the person to make a piece of art following your directions. For example, ask them to look through magazines and cut out several pictures (for example, food, clothing, and famous people) that they would like to use to create the piece of art. After they cut the pictures out, ask them to tape or glue the pictures on the large piece of paper in whatever arrangement they prefer. Once they attach the pictures to the blank piece of paper, ask the person to use the colored pencils or markers to write meaningful words throughout and around the blank spaces to enhance the piece of art. When they complete the task, ask them to sign the art, as artists do. Be sure to engage them in conversation about the collage that they created (for example, ask them to describe it, why they chose certain pictures).

Alternate example: You can modify this activity and strategy to include painting an original piece. Provide the person with the tools to paint (canvas paper, acrylic paints, and fine-point color markers). For example, first ask the person to view a variety of paintings from a book or online. After you and your loved one view the paintings, ask them to pick one painting that motivates and is meaningful to them. Once they choose a painting, ask them to study, review, and comment on it. You will then remove the painting from view and ask the person to paint their version of it. If the person requires the painting to be in view, you may leave the painting there as a cue; however, the outcome would then be a re-creation of the painting.

Your turn: Think about the person in your care and create an alternative activity and strategy that best meets the interests and needs of that person.

TABLE 8.1. *The Forms of Expression and Participation for an Art Activity*

APPRECIATION	RE-CREATION	CREATION
Activity: Viewing paintings in a local art museum or online	**Activity:** Copying line drawings or pictures of functional objects that are part of a person's daily routine	**Activity:** Making an art collage
Strategy: While the person is viewing each painting, ask closed (yes or no) and open-ended questions (How does it make you feel?)	**Strategy:** Show the person the picture you want them to name and draw (copy while in view)	**Strategy:** Provide the person with a large piece of canvas art paper (16″ × 20″, or tape four 8″ × 10″ pieces of paper together), colored pencils, markers, scissors, tape, glue, and several magazines
Goal: Improve verbal and gestural commenting	**Goal:** Improve word finding and ability to convey a message	**Goal:** Improve following directions, writing, word retrieval, recall, and organization skills

MUSIC
Unleashing the Inner Sinatra

Appreciation

Activity: Listening to a classical, doo-wop, rock, pop, or another favorite type of music

Strategy: While the person is listening to the music, ask the following questions:

> Is it a happy song?
> Is it a sad song?
> What instruments do you hear?
> Who is singing?
> How does it make you feel?

Alternate example: You can change this activity and strategy to include other types of music, such as Broadway musicals, operas, or symphonies that may interest the person. You can modify questions to suit the type of music.

Your turn: Think about the person in your care and create an alternative activity and strategy that best meets the interests and needs of that person.

Re-creation

Activity: Sing along

Strategy: Search the web for online karaoke songs. Let the person choose the song. It should have an upbeat rhythm and repetitive lyrics (for example, "Sweet Caroline," by Neil Diamond; "I Love Rock 'n' Roll," by Joan Jett; or "Mamma Mia," by ABBA). Play the song and ask the person to sing along with the words. If needed, write out the words of the song. Initially, you will find that you must sing along with the person to help them. With time and practice, eventually the person should sing portions of the song independently.

Alternate example: You can change this activity and strategy to include portions of a Broadway musical. The person can choose a favorite musical, and you can determine the songs or portions of the musical that you will use for the activity. You would follow a similar format in the previous example and pick the songs with lyrics written out for the person to follow when singing. Watching a video of the musical song would also be helpful but is not required.

Your turn: Think about the person that is in your care and create an alternative activity and strategy that best meets the interests and needs of that person.

Creation

Activity: Writing new lyrics to an existing melody or song.

Strategy: Find a song that has a strong and repetitive melody and is very familiar to your loved one and others (for example, "We Are the World," by Michael Jackson and Lionel Richie). To assist the person, you can use a karaoke version with vocals removed, or a melody or song written without vocals. Have the person listen to a portion of the song that is repetitive or considered to be the chorus and ask them to write new words to the melody that are meaningful (for example, "You Can't Hurry Speech" to the tune of "You Can't Hurry Love," by the Supremes). If the person cannot write, you can write the words for the person. For example, a person who is living with Parkinson's disease or aphasia may use words to talk about life experiences or what it's like living with Parkinson's disease or aphasia and replace the words in the song with the new words.

Alternate example: If your loved one plays a musical instrument, you can modify this activity and strategy. Have them play a melody on the instrument and add words to that melody, as you write the words down. Finding the words may be a challenge for that person, but the melody created from the instrument may help the words come out. You may need to cue them to their specific environment, situation, or family to help them find words to go with the melody. For example, if you tell the person to think of their children or pets, this may help the person remember words of their children or pets to add to the melody.

Your turn: Think about the person in your care and create an alternative activity and strategy that best meets the interests and needs of that person.

TABLE 8.2. *The Forms of Expression and Participation for a Music Activity*

APPRECIATION	RE-CREATION	CREATION
Activity: Listening to a classical, doo-wop, rock, pop, or another favorite type of music	**Activity:** Sing along	**Activity:** Writing new lyrics to an existing melody or song
Strategy: While the person is listening to the music, ask closed and open-ended questions	**Strategy:** Search the web for online karaoke songs; let the person choose the song	**Strategy:** Find a song that has a strong and repetitive melody and is liked and very familiar
Goal: Improve verbal and gestural commenting	**Goal:** Improve verbalizations	**Goal:** Improve recall, word finding, and writing

DANCE
Unleashing the Inner Astaire

Appreciation

Activity: Viewing a dance routine of a waltz, rumba, foxtrot, jitterbug, or other favorite type of dance.

Strategy: While the person is watching the dance routine, ask the following questions:

> Is it a slow dance?
> Is it a fast dance?
> Are the dancers good?
> What is the dance?
> What type of music are they dancing too?
> How would you describe the costumes
>   they are wearing?
> Overall, what do you think of the dance?

Alternate example: You can modify this activity and strategy to include other types of dance, such as ballet, modern, and jazz that may interest the person. You can change questions to suit the type of dance.

Your turn: Think about the person in your care and create an alternative activity and strategy that best meets the interests and needs of that person.

Re-creation

Activity: Dance along

Strategy: If the person or you have a background in dancing and previously enjoyed dancing, start here. To improve recall and following directions, teach or reteach the person a specific dance. Choose a dance that is easy to learn (for example, foxtrot, swing, or cha cha). When engaging the person in the activity, ask them to follow your directions for a portion of the dance by competing the steps to the dance. If your loved one cannot follow the directions, you may need to have them say or write the directions down, or you may need to say the directions while modeling the steps to the dance, as the person completes the dance with you. After they successfully complete following the directions and portion of the dance, ask them to comment aloud or in writing on what they thought about that portion of the dance and what they could improve.

Alternate example: You can change this activity and strategy if the person is a beginner and is new to dance by using line dancing (for example, the Electric Slide, the Cowboy Hustle, or Hokey Pokey). Have the person dance along with you, and if possible, play a video of the dance and song that accompanies the dance movements.

Your turn: Think about the person in your care and create an alternative activity and strategy that best meets the interests and needs of that person.

Creation

Activity: Developing new dance moves to an existing song

Strategy: Find a song that has a strong and repetitive melody and is familiar to the person. To assist them, you can use a karaoke version with vocals removed, or a song with no lyrics. To improve listening, recall, following directions, and writing skills, have the person listen to a portion of the song that is repetitive or considered to be the chorus, and ask them to write dance steps or body movements (for example, step touch step, right hand raised, then left hand raised, then both hands raised, and clap). If the person cannot write, you can write the steps for them.

Alternate example: You can change and implement this activity and strategy with someone in a wheelchair by using his or her upper body or movement of the wheelchair during the dance routine.

Your turn: Think about the person in your care and create an alternative activity and strategy that best meets the interests and needs of that person.

TABLE 8.3. *The Forms of Expression and Participation for a Dance Activity*

APPRECIATION	RE-CREATION	CREATION
Activity: Viewing a dance routine of a waltz, rumba, foxtrot, jitterbug, or other favorite type of dance	**Activity:** Dance along	**Activity:** Developing new dance moves to an existing song
Strategy: While the person is watching the dance routine, ask closed and open-ended questions	**Strategy:** If the person or caregiver has a background in dancing and previously enjoyed dancing, start here	**Strategy:** Find a song that has a strong and repetitive melody and is liked and familiar to the person
Goal: Improve verbal and gestural commenting	**Goal:** Improve recall and following directions	**Goal:** Improve listening, recall, following directions, and writing skills

ACTING
Unleashing the Inner Streep

Appreciation

Activity: Viewing a clip from a favorite television show or movie

Strategy: During or after the person watches the clip, ask the following questions:

> Is it a comedy? If so, what is funny about it?
> Is it a drama? If so, what is sad about it?
> What's the name of the show?
> Who are the actors?
> What's the show about?

Alternate example: You can change this activity and strategy to include other types of acting (for example, documentaries, news stories, and theatrical productions) that may interest the person. You can modify questions to suit the specific type of acting.

Your turn: Think about the person in your care and create an alternative activity and strategy that best meets the interests and needs of that person.

Re-creation

Activity: Orally reading and acting out short scripts or plays

Strategy: Find short scripts or plays created for adults through an online venue or the library. Two-person scripts are most appropriate for this activity. Once found, provide the person with the script and ask them to pick a role that is most suited or motivating to them. You will do the same. An oral reading of the script then begins. While the person is reading the part, prompt for the use of good speaking skills. For example, ask them to use the skills learned in speech therapy, such as using good breath support when speaking ("Make sure you take a deep breath before you speak"), overpronunciation of each sound in words ("Concentrate on moving your lips and tongue when you are speaking"), and speaking at a loud enough volume so that the listener will hear ("Speak loud enough so that the person at the other end of the room can hear you"). Point out to the person that these basic good speaking skills will help listeners better understand. Observe the person reading the role and provide feedback regarding pronunciation, volume, and breath support (see chapters 2 and 3).

Alternate example: You can change this activity and strategy to include an increased number of participants when visiting immediate or extended family. For example, you can all gather in the living room and put on a play. Give all the family members a character to act out, and if possible, give the person with communication impairment the lead, so they can interact with all the actors.

Your turn: Think about the person in your care and create an alternative activity and strategy that best meets the interests and needs of that person.

Creation

Activity: Rearranging a script

Strategy: Find short scripts or plays created for adults through an online venue or library. Once you find the script or play, ask your loved one to take a portion of the script and rewrite it with a different outcome or focus. If the person cannot write, you can write for them. For example, ask them to provide a different ending to the script. Ask them to rewrite the description of their character. For example, they could change a role in the script to someone who recently had a stroke. This can give the person an opportunity to express feelings about how they are coping or living with disability. You can also use the rewritten version of the script to improve the person's speaking skills, such as volume and pronunciation, through orally reading and acting out the rewrite.

Alternate example: You can change this activity and strategy to include mime and gestures, such as through the classic game of Charades. Think of ideas that fall into the category of a movie (such as *The Godfather*), book (such as *To Kill a Mockingbird*), character (such as Superman), actions (such as playing a specific sport), or something from another category chosen by the players. An important tip is to make sure every single person will be able to guess a word, and that words used are familiar to them. Put these ideas on slips of paper and place them into a container. Then have someone draw a slip and show it to the person who then must act out the charade's idea. Using gestures or acting abilities, the person must make the others correctly guess the idea. You may need to assist your loved one as needed. For example, you may need to ask the person to reread the word associated with the gesture.

Your turn: Think about the person in your care and create an alternative activity and strategy that best meets the interests and needs of that person. Consider goals that are specific to the person.

TABLE 8.4. *The Forms of Expression and Participation for an Acting Activity*

APPRECIATION	RE-CREATION	CREATION
Activity: Viewing a clip from a favorite television show or movie	**Activity:** Orally reading and acting out short scripts or plays	**Activity:** Rearranging a script
Strategy: While the person is viewing each clip, ask closed and open-ended questions	**Strategy:** Find short scripts or plays created for adults through an online venue or the library; two-person scripts are most appropriate for this activity	**Strategy:** Find short scripts or plays created for adults and ask the person to take a portion of the script and rewrite it with a different outcome or focus
Goal: Improve verbal and gestural commenting	**Goal:** Improve speaking skills	**Goal:** Improve recall, word finding, reading comprehension, and writing

As the caregiver, consider opportunities for communication that occur before and after the activity, not just during the activity. Before and after opportunities provide increased time for reflection and communication, whether in appreciation, re-creation, or creation. For example, prior to engaging in an art activity that includes visiting a museum, you might discuss with the person the specific museum you will visit, review a map of the museum, and discuss specific areas in the building. After the activity, you can take the person to the museum gift shop and discuss the various souvenirs available for sale, and if you purchase a souvenir, you can involve the person with the sales transaction and communicating with the store salesperson. As an additional example, prior to engaging in an acting activity that includes choosing a script to act out, you can ask the person what types of plays or scripts they enjoy. If the choice is comedy or drama, help select the script and discuss the character in the script this person may want to play. After the person acts out the character in the script, ask what they thought of the acting performance. Give your loved one an opportunity to reflect on the skills learned in speech therapy. You could ask questions like, "Did you take a deep breath before speaking?" "Did you concentrate on moving your lips and tongue when speaking?" or "Did you speak loudly enough?" These examples of before and after opportunities provide you with samples that you can adapt to other arts activities within the areas of art, music, dance, or acting. The important concept to keep in mind is that the before and after encounters will provide the person with as many opportunities as possible to communicate.

Personal Examples of How the Arts Have Helped Patients with Communication Disorders

The following three examples include specific activities I have used at Nova Southeastern University (NSU) Speech-Language Pathology Clinic to improve communication, socialization, and quality of life in adults living with communication disorders. These examples include (1) painting, drawing, coloring, and mixed-media design; (2) music, singing, and dancing; and (3) writing a script, singing, and acting. Specific treatment techniques using the arts took place while the people with communication impairments were also receiving individual or group speech therapy. I used treatment techniques with adults with communication disorders over time to produce a functional result that showcased their talents and, most importantly, progressed with treatment goals. A home program implemented with the patients and caregivers from week to week was a key element in achieving a positive result. The planning process included a weekly group treatment session, an individual treatment session for some, and a home program implemented with the caregiver for both group and individual treatment.

Example 1: Art through the Hemispheres

I used elements of painting, drawing, coloring, and collage in working with persons with aphasia and their caregivers. As discussed in chapter 5, aphasia is a communication disorder caused by damage to the parts of the brain used for speech and language. These individuals created works of art that were on display at an art gallery opening held at the NSU Speech-Language Pathology Clinic. The title of the event was "Art through the Hemispheres." The functional outcome and result of the event included the aphasia group patients and caregivers presenting their art gallery pieces. The patients spoke about the benefits of using art to improve communication, socialization, and quality of life. This event gave the patients a platform to "unleash their inner Picasso."

Example 2: Dancing with the Aphasia Group Stars

Other treatment strategies I used with aphasia group patients and their caregivers incorporated the use of artistic expression through music, singing, and dancing. Two of the aphasia patients and their spouses were previously ballroom dancers, and they came to life on the dance floor. They moved, sang, followed directions, and smiled as if they were Fred Astaire and Ginger Rogers. It struck me that learning the waltz and foxtrot could nudge other aphasic patients out of their shells and move them to interact and talk to others. When the patients and their caregivers agreed to give it a go, the Dancing with the Aphasia Group Stars show, modeled after the television show *Dancing with the Stars*, was born. The seasoned ballroom-dancer patients and their caregivers taught the other group members the dance steps. The patients learned to follow specific instructions and use words tailored to their needs while they were learning to dance. The patients and their caregivers all took part in Dancing with the Aphasia Group Stars. During one dance routine, a nonverbal patient and her spouse were dancing a foxtrot to "Fly Me to the Moon," by Frank Sinatra. While dancing, the patient sang every word to the song as her spouse and the audience beamed. The judges were two speech-language pathologists and one occupational therapist. The first- through third-place winners received trophies. One patient's spouse stood up to share her ultimate praise for the show and the care received by her and her husband, saying, "This experience changed our lives. Now my husband is talking more and is more engaged."

Example 3: The Parkinson's Monologues

Treatment strategies I used with Parkinson's group patients incorporated the use of artistic expression through writing scripts and songs and then acting and singing. To give these individuals the opportunity to tell their stories of living with their disease, they wrote and later performed dramatic monologues. The idea came as an ode to the *Vagina Monologues*, an off-Broadway play in New York that inspired my artistic treatment approach. I envisioned a play of monologues about the Parkinson's experience. Parkinson's disease is a progressive nervous system disorder that affects communication, cognition, and movement. Some symptoms include speech and writing changes, rigid and slowed movement, and tremors. The result was The Parkinson's Players, a group of adults who took part in a weekly support and treatment group that not only helped them deal with their struggles with speech and language, but also turned them into actors. By the time the players rehearsed and eventually stood on a stage to deliver their monologues to a 150-person audience, they were speaking with clarity, conviction, and confidence, unleashing their inner Meryl Streep.

What Are the Important Take-Home Points in This Chapter?

- Art, music, dance, and acting stimulate the entire brain, while increasing motivation and socialization.

- Forms of artistic treatment and activities are not just for the person with a communication impairment, but also for caregivers, family, and friends who interact with the person.

- The main goal is to make activities fun, engaging, motivating, and functional for the individual with a communication impairment, based on their hobbies and interests.

- Determine what the person's artistic interests were in the past, before their impairment.

- You can find materials for these activities in your home, local library, or online (for example, Pinterest, Google, or YouTube).

- Consultation and collaboration with an arts-based therapist (e.g., music therapist or drama therapist) can further enhance improvement with communication, especially if the individual responds well to the arts.

This chapter provides you, the caregiver, with knowledge, examples, and tools to incorporate the arts into your loved one's life. Take the leap and use the arts as an exciting and creative tool to empower the person you care for. And who knows, the person you care for may just unleash their inner Pablo Picasso, Frank Sinatra, Fred Astaire, or Meryl Streep!

REFERENCES

Boster, J. B., McCarthy, J. W., Spitzley, A., Corso, C., Castle, T., & Jewell, A. (2018). Using art to improve social and participation outcomes for individuals with communication disorders: A systematic review. Paper presented at the American Speech-Language-Hearing Association (ASHA) Convention, November 15–17, 2018, Boston, Massachusetts.

Hajjar, D. J., & McCarthy, J. W. (2014). Music has positive effects for individuals with neurological speech and language disorders, but questions remain regarding type, timing, and fidelity of treatment. *Evidence-Based Communication Assessment and Intervention*, 8(3), 116–23. https://doi.org/10.1080/17 489539.2014.1001548.

RESOURCES

Local Public Library

Google: https://www.google.com

Pinterest: https://www.pinterest.com

Search Terms

   Art: collage, drawings, mixed media, paintings, sculpture

   Music: Broadway musicals, karaoke, opera, pop, symphonics

   Dance: ballroom, line dancing

   Acting: charades, mime, movies, play scripts for adults, television

ABOUT THE AUTHOR

Dr. Frederick DiCarlo is an Associate Professor in the Department of Speech-Language Pathology at Nova Southeastern University (NSU), Florida. He has twenty-five years of experience assessing and treating adults with neurogenic communication disorders in various academic and medical settings. Dr. DiCarlo's lifelong passion for the arts inspired him to study fine arts–dance in his undergraduate program. Dr. DiCarlo supervises a Parkinson's support group and individual and group aphasia treatment at NSU. His creative incorporation of acting, dance, music, and painting into his individual and group treatment sessions has earned him accolades in the American Speech-Language-Hearing Association (ASHA) *Leader* and from Channel 10 news in Miami, Florida. Recently, due to the Covid-19 pandemic, Dr. DiCarlo established a telepractice presence using the arts for his patients with aphasia and Parkinson's disease.

About the Editors

Dr. Barbara O'Connor Wells

Dr. Barbara O'Connor Wells is an Associate Professor and Clinical Supervisor in the Department of Speech-Language Pathology at Nova Southeastern University (NSU). She received her BA in Speech Pathology and Audiology and her MA in Speech-Language Pathology from St. John's University, New York, and her PhD in Speech-Language-Hearing Sciences from the Graduate Center of the City University of New York (CUNY). She teaches coursework and supervises individual and group treatment sessions in the areas of dysphagia, motor speech, and adult language disorders at NSU.

Dr. O'Connor Wells is certified by the American Speech-Language-Hearing Association (ASHA) and has twenty-five years of experience in acute, subacute, long-term, and homecare rehabilitation of adult neurogenic communication, cognition, and swallowing disorders. She is licensed in both Florida and New York and maintains active membership in the Florida Association of Speech-Language Pathologists and Audiologists (FLASHA), the New York State Speech-Language-Hearing Association (NYSSLHA), and the Irish Association of Speech and Language Therapists (IASLT). Her clinical experiences have traversed the lifespan, from infants to older adults, and she has also practiced clinically in schools and private practice settings. Prior to NSU, Dr. O'Connor Wells was an Instructor in the Communication Sciences Program at Hunter College, CUNY. Her primary research and clinical interests include dysphagia, aphasia in monolingual and bilingual populations, aphasia in Spanish speakers, and the aging brain. She has several journal article and book chapter publications in scholarly journals, including *Clinical Linguistics and Phonetics*, *Brain and Language*, and *Topics in Geriatric Medicine*, and has a long history of national and international conference presentations in locations such as Florida, Boston, New York, Spain, Germany, Cyprus, and Oxford University. She is currently involved in several research projects at NSU: swallowing disorders in individuals with Chagas disease in South America, viscosity of the Varibar barium product used during the modified barium swallow study, aphasia in Spanish speakers, and bilingual aphasia treatment.

Dr. Connie K. Porcaro

Dr. Connie Porcaro is an Associate Professor in the Department of Communication Sciences and Disorders at Florida Atlantic University (FAU). She received her BA in Communication Sciences and Disorders from the University of South Dakota, her MA in Speech Pathology from the University of Northern Colorado, and her PhD in Speech and Hearing Sciences from the University of Arizona. Dr. Porcaro instructs courses at FAU covering voice, speech, and swallowing disorders in adults. She lectures annually for the FAU Charles E. Schmidt College of Medicine on the topics of adult neurogenic communication disorders.

Dr. Porcaro is certified by the American Speech-Language-Hearing Association (ASHA) and has worked as a speech-language pathologist for more than twenty-five years with clients of all ages. Her primary area of research has focused on intelligibility in patients with speech and voice disorders and how speakers can improve communication with their listeners. She has published research articles in top journals, including the *American Journal of Speech-Language Pathology* and the *International Journal of Speech-Language Pathology*. Dr. Porcaro is a frequent presenter at the annual ASHA convention and often presents for state association conventions as an invited speaker. She is an active member of the Leadership Team Professional Development Subcommittee for the ASHA Special Interest Group on Neurophysiology and Neurogenic Speech and Language Disorders. She has received grant funding from the FAU Healthy Aging Research Initiative to investigate voice and swallowing changes in healthy elderly participants. Dr. Porcaro has received grant funding from the Parkinson Voice Project to facilitate training for graduate students who provide free speech therapy for individuals with Parkinson's disease.

Appendix A

Voice Illustration

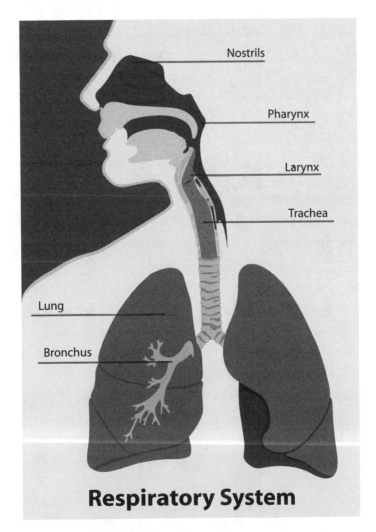

Appendix B

Alphabet Board Example

A	B	C	D	Hello	Good-bye
E	F	G	H	Yes	No
I	J	K	L	M	N
O	P	Q	R	S	T
U	V	W	X	Y	Z
Drink	Food	Bed	Pain	Help	Stop

Appendix C

Swallowing Illustration

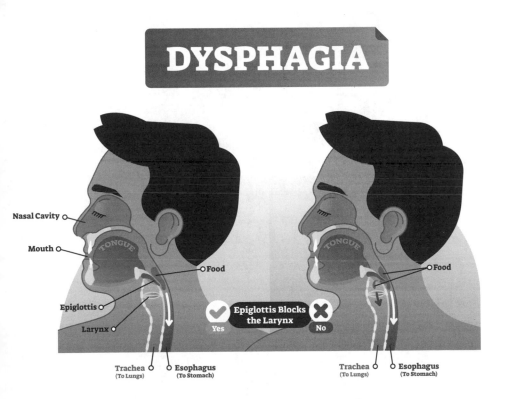

Appendix D

Brain Illustration

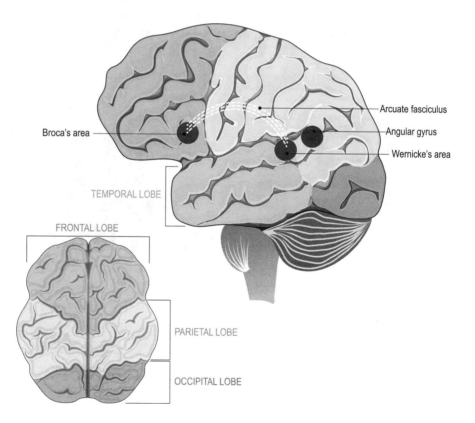

Index